Wonderful feeling of Tai Chi spirit

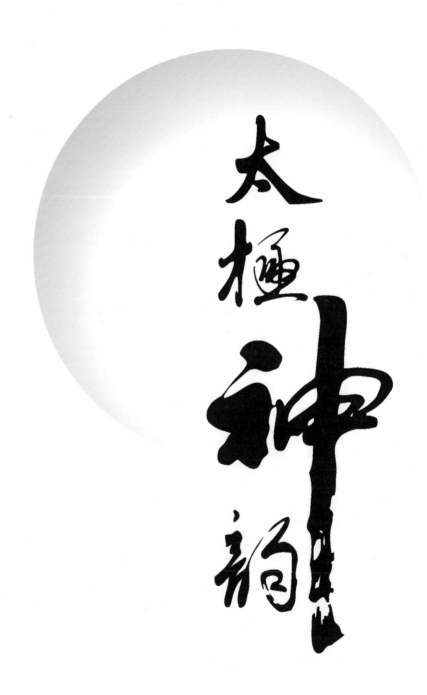

Hand written calligraphy
by Grandmaster
Chen Zhenglei in China

Tai Chi
For Health

Written by Grandmaster Chen Zhenglei and Master Liming Yue

Co-authors: Dan Chisholm, Tim Birch, Steven Burton, Nick Taylor
Anthony Ruston and Bill Wilkinson

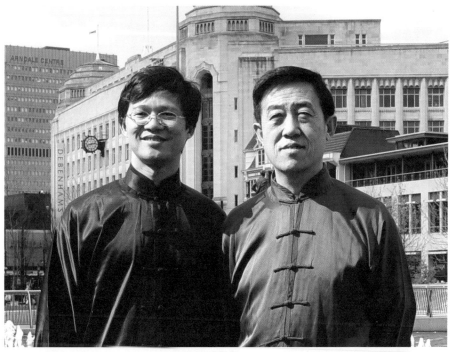

Grandmaster Chen Zhenglei and Master Liming Yue

This book was written by Grandmaster Chen Zhenglei and Master Liming Yue over a two and a half year period. It is recognized by the International Tai Chi Festival committee and the Chinese Martial Arts Association in China. It is a highly recommended instructional book to the Tai Chi practitioner across the world. The book was officially released at the opening ceremony of the International Taijiquan (Tai Chi) Festival and the 3rd International Taijiquan Exchange Competition in Jiaozuo City, Chinese August 2005, which is hosted by the Chinese Martial Arts Association and the Henan Province Sports Council.

Disclaimer

The views expressed in the book are the views of the writers and are not necessarily in accordance with the views of the Publisher, the Chen Style Tai Chi Centre.

© Copyright 2005 by:

Master Liming Yue, Chen Style Tai Chi Centre U.K.

ISBN: 1-94719120 (Hardback edition); 1-94719112 (Paperback edition)

Published by: Chen Style Tai Chi Centre, U.K.

Tel: +44 (0) 161 2737138

Fax: +44(0) 161 2744967

E-Mail: info@taichicentre.com

Web site: www.taichicentre.com

Address: PO Box 137, Manchester, M60 1WL, U.K.

Date of Release: 20/08/2005 (at the Tai Chi Festival in China)

Printed by: Henan Tianxing Shangpin Visual & Media Ltd.

Amount of copies: 5,000 (paperback 3,000 and hardback 2,000)

Cover Designer: Master Liming Yue, Duan Yingying

Book Editor: Master Liming Yue, Duan Yingying

Photography by: Master Liming Yue, Mr. Yongsheng Yue

Proof Readers: Chen Xiaobin, Bill Wilkinson, Linda Wilkinson, Geoff Leversedge, Sue Johnson, Ploutarchos Vlachopoulos, Peter Donaldson, Nick Taylor, Dan Chisholm, Anthony Rushton, Alastair Macgillivray, Tim Birch, Steven Burton, John Bolwell. Cemil Egeli, Mark Guggiari, Aamir Rafi, Bruce Li, Gillian Egeli and Diana Dicker.

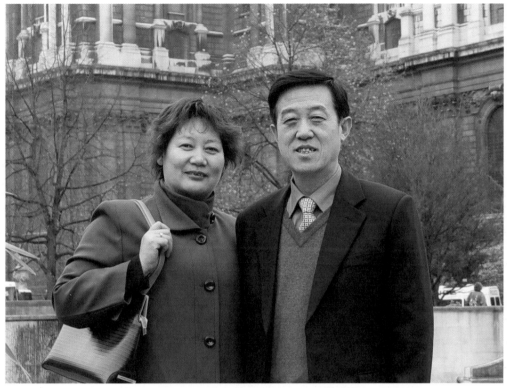

Grandmaster Chen Zhenglei and his wife – Mrs. Lu Lili visit London, April 2003.

Grandmaster Chen Zhenglei, 11th generation Head of Chen Style Taijiquan, 19th Generation of the Chen family.

Grandmaster Chen Zhenglei is ranked as one of the Top Ten Martial Arts Grandmasters in China and is honored for numerous contributions to Martial Arts by the Chinese State Sports Council.

Chen Style Family Taijiquan is the original form from which all modern forms of Taijiquan have developed – come and drink from the source.

The ancient Yin Yang philosophy is over 2000 years old and comes from the I Ching – Book of Changes. Around 350 years ago, the 9th generation Chen family Grandmaster Chen Wangting created the original and authentic Chen Style Tai Chi hand form movements, weapon forms and routines, push hands and Qigong exercises. They combine Yin and Yang philosophy with Chinese Martial Arts movements and breathing techniques. Originally these wonderful powerful Martial Arts exercises were a carefully guarded secret, kept in the Chen village, Wen county, Henan Province, P.R. China, and only passed on to family members. This is the first time that the whole series of health exercises has been opened up and made available worldwide by the 19th generation Chen family representative, Grandmaster Chen Zhenglei.

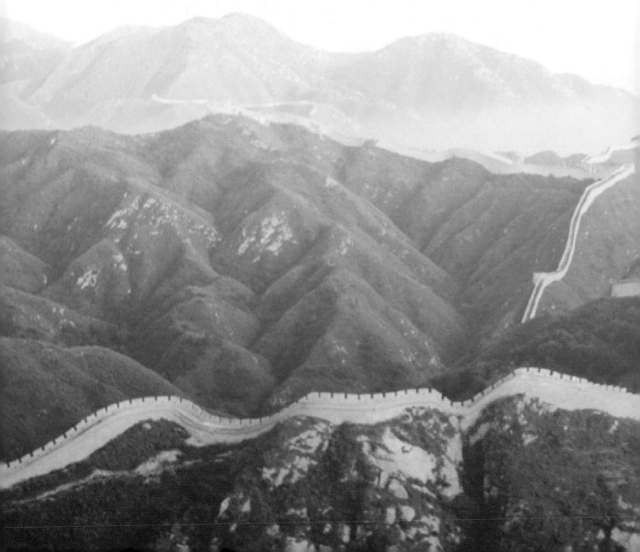

太極願世界和平

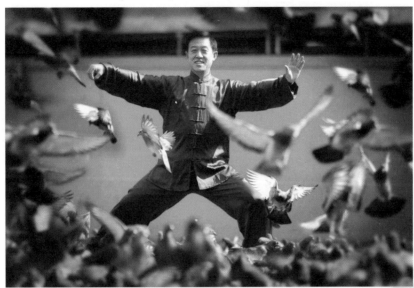

Tai Chi brings peace and health to the world
Photographed and published by Manchester Evening News 2003

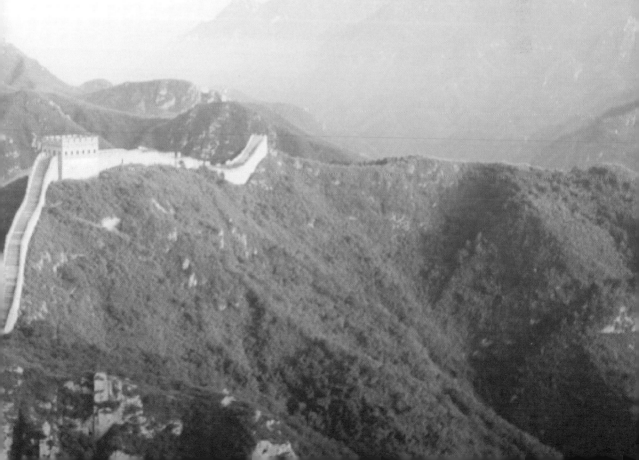

Table of Contents

The end

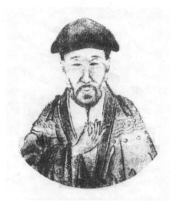

太極拳創始人陳王庭遺像（1600-1680）

Grandmaster Chen Wangting – The
founder of Chen Style Tai Chi and seventh
generation of Chen Family (1600 1680).

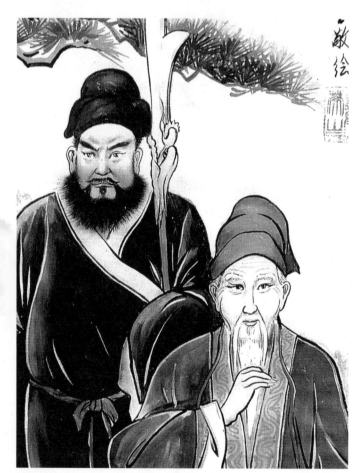

Grandmaster Chen Wangting with his senior student
Jiang Fa (stand behind)

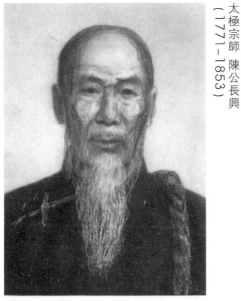

太極宗師 陳公長興
（1771-1853）

Grandmaster Chen Changxing – the fourteenth generation of Chen Family and the Sifu of Yang Luchan, who is the founder of Yang Style Tai Chi.

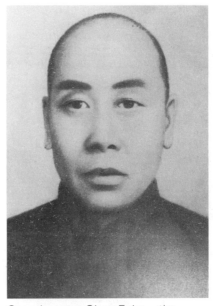

陳發科老師
陳氏十七世、太極拳第九代傳人
（1887-1957）

Grandmaster Chen Fake – the seventeenth generation of Chen Family and the final founder of Xinjia – 83 Form and Cannon Fist.

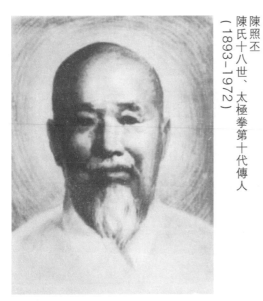

陳照丕
陳氏十八世、太極拳第十代傳人
（1893-1972）

Grandmaster Chen Zhaopi – the 18th Generation of Chen Family and the primary Sifu of Grandmaster Chen Zhenglei.

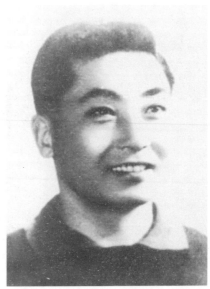

陳照奎
陳氏十八世、太極拳第十代傳人
（1928-1981）

Grandmaster Chen Zhaokui – the 18th Generation of Chen Family.

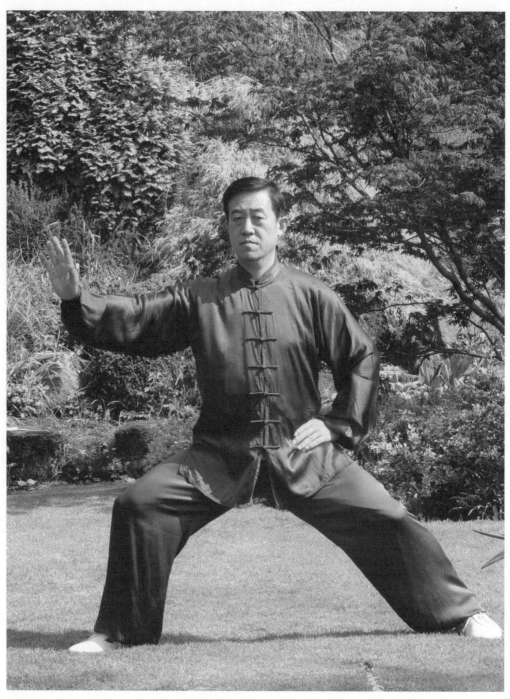

Lazy About Tying Coat posture taken in a park in Manchester, UK 2003.
Photograph taken by Master Liming Yue.

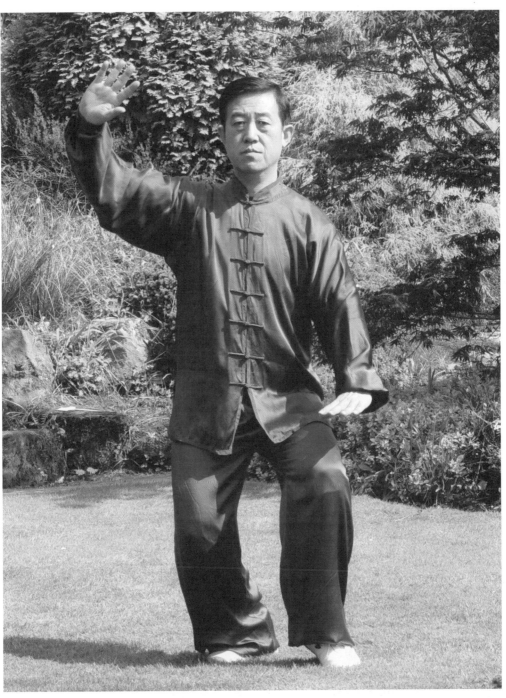

White Crane Spreads its Wings.

太極
養生功

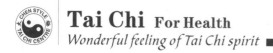

Tai Chi For Health
Wonderful feeling of Tai Chi spirit

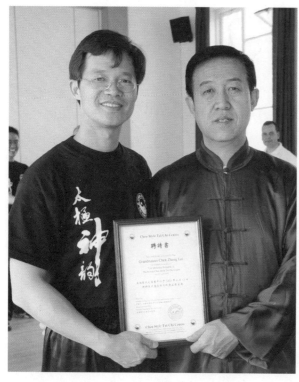

太極揚天下

Grandmaster Chen Zhenglei accepts Honorary Presidency of the Chen Style Tai Chi Centre UK in 2003.

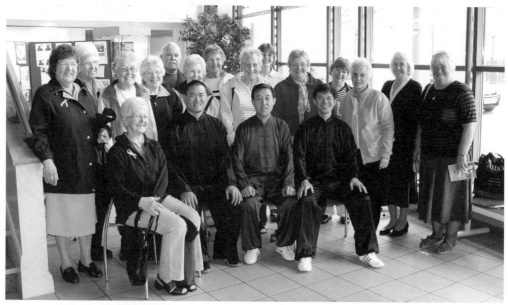

Grandmaster Chen Zhenglei with Master Liming Yue and Wang Haijun meet a group of students from AGE Concern, Ashton – U – Lyne, Manchester, UK 2003.

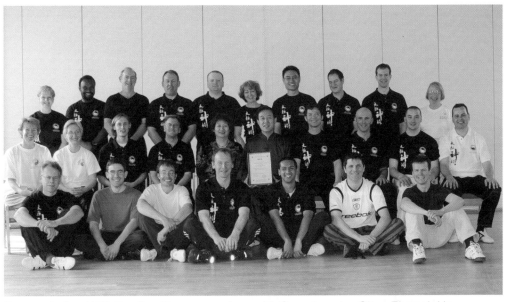

Group photo of Silk Reeling Energy seminar with Grandmaster Chen Zhenglei in Manchester, UK 2003.

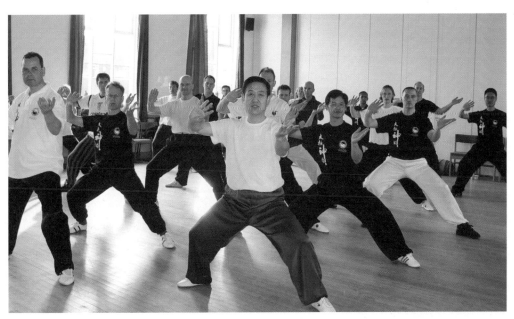

83 Form seminar with Grandmaster Chen Zhenglei in Manchester, UK 2003.

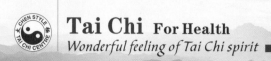

Tai Chi For Health
Wonderful feeling of Tai Chi spirit

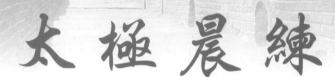

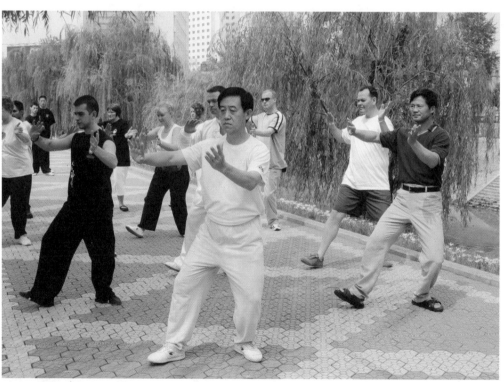

Morning practice in the park in China during the China Trip 2004 organized by Chen Style Tai Chi Centre UK. Training led by Grandmaster Chen Zhenglei.

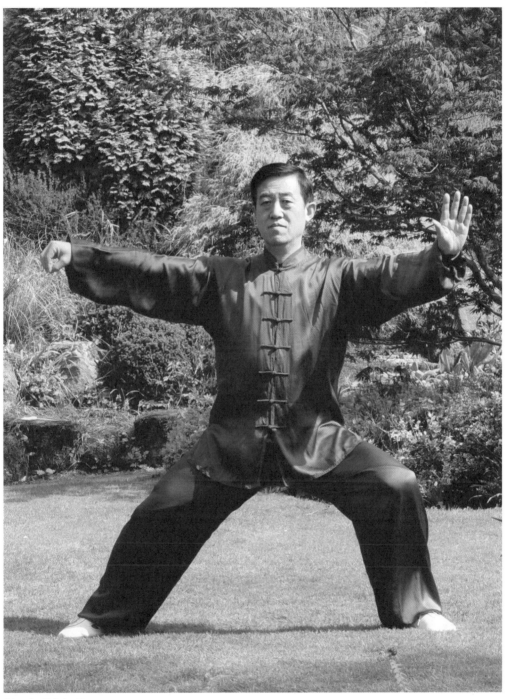

Single Whip Posture.

太極
養生功

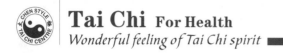
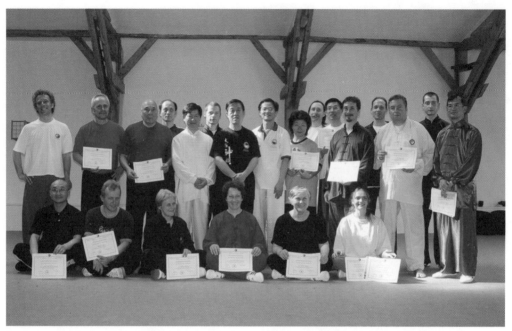

Seminars in Paris, France 2003 in Dr. Jian Niujun Tai Chi and Qigong College.

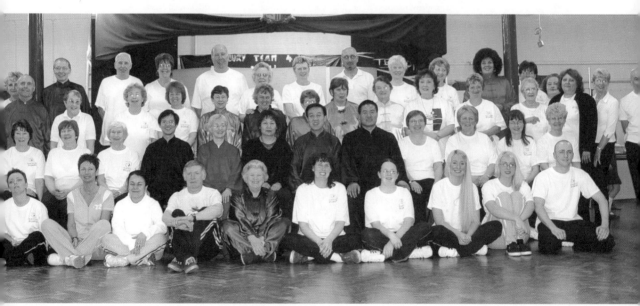

UK visit to Chen Style Tai Chi College in Bury, Greater Manchester 2003 by Grandmaster Chen Zhenglei and his wife – Lu Lili.

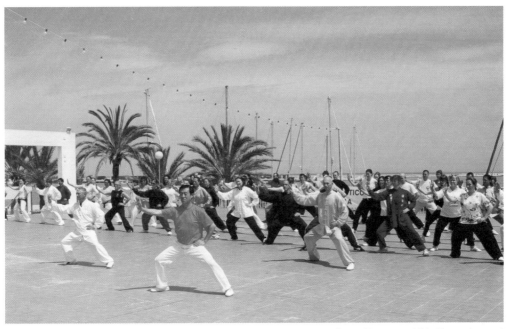

Residential seminars in Denia, Spain 2004 with attendants from France, UK, Canada and local students from Spain.

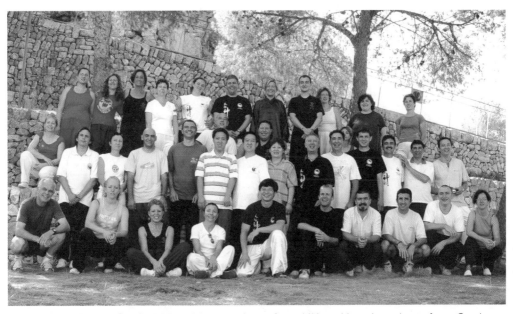

Seminars in Denia, Spain 2005 with attendants from UK and local students from Spain.

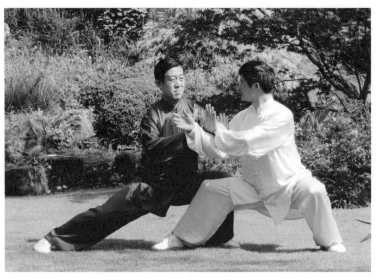

Push Hands by Grandmaster Chen Zhenglei and Master Liming Yue in Manchester, UK 2003.

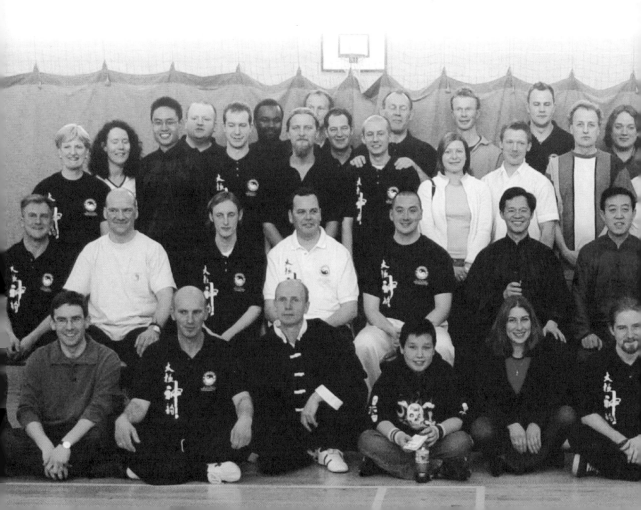

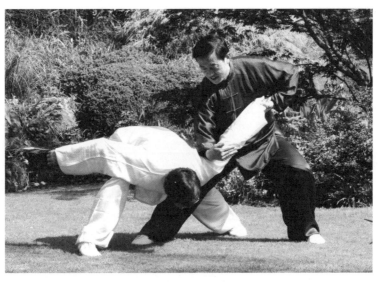

Arm lock application by Grandmaster Chen Zhenglei and
Master Liming Yue in Manchester UK 2003.

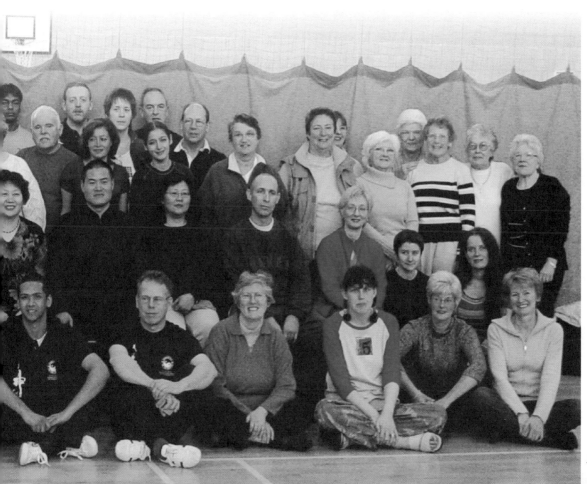

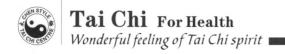

Foreword

by Grandmaster Chen Zhenglei

Economic progress, social reforms, improvement in living standards and greater automation in people's daily working lives have all contributed to a general reduction in the levels of physical exercise and fitness. As activity and exercise decrease, physical and mental health as well as general well-being begin to deteriorate. More and more people are turning to practices like "Wushu" and "Qigong" to try to redress this imbalance in their lives.

For a long time Taijiquan has been held in very high esteem by many Chinese people. In the last century, it has become more popular in the rest of the world because of its health enhancing and self-defence qualities. "Taijiquan" strengthens bones and muscles, regulates "Jingluo" (the body's main energy channels), keeps in balance the nervous system and helps prevent the onset of disease. Personally, I have practiced "Taijiquan" since I was a child. I have first hand, personal experience of its health benefits and particularly of "Qigong". For centuries, the special benefits and practice of "Qigong" were closely guarded secrets inside the Chen village where I was born. Even though it has seldom spread outside of my village, I now wish to share its secrets and recommend its practice to everyone who is interested in its health enhancing properties.

"Taiji", born out of "Wuji", was divided into "Liangyi", changed into "Sancai", then "Sixiang", ultimately evolving into the eight Diagrams and then to Infinity. "Qigong" is the new term, which has appeared in recent years and is synonymous with internal energy "Kung Fu". The internal energy aspects of "Qigong" are at the very heart of "Taijiquan". Its purpose is to understand and learn how to collect, develop and increase internal energy. This internal energy is then retained in the "Dantian", is upgraded to a

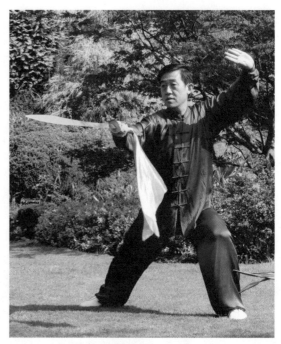

Chen Style Tai Chi Sabre posture.

spiritual level and then released back to non-existence. The development of physical energy into spiritual energy allows space, earth, body and nature to exist as one and is the ultimate goal of "Qigong".

There are some old Chinese sayings, "Look after the roots and the leaves and flowers will grow healthy." "If plenty of water is feeding the stream, the stream will last longer and go further." "Tai Chi" internal energy "Qigong" is based on the same principles of looking after and taking care of individual's sources of energy. With this book, I wish to share and introduce to all people interested in "Taiji", Chen

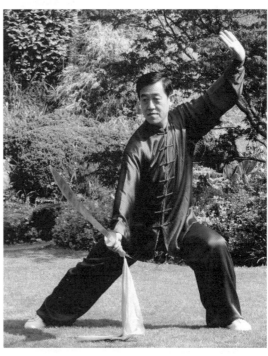

Chen Style Tai Chi Sabre posture.

Style Taijiquan for health, the "Taiji" skills of internal energy and The 18 forms of Chen Style "Taijiquan". In this way, everyone can begin to understand and to realize the physical health and mental benefits to be gained from regular practice of "Taijiquan".

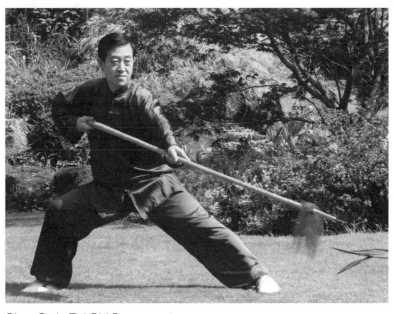

Chen Style Tai Chi Spear posture.

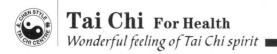

Guidelines for using this book

This book offers an easygoing introduction to Chen Style Tai Chi. An authentic, comprehensive reference book for the specific style of Tai Chi, the content also pays particular attention to the health benefits avilaible to students. There are also two volumes of instructional DVDs/Videos available from the Chen Style Tai Chi Centre UK which accompany this book. Silk Reeling Energy and Tai Chi 18 Short Form. These DVDs are available from the online shop: www.shop.taichicentre.com

For better understanding, readers may wish to refer to the direct insights from first person accounts. See Chapter 6: Interviews with Practitioners. Whether you decide to read this book in a linear fashion or not, readers are advised that a method of continual reference will prove the most beneficial. Practitioners of Chen Style Tai Chi undertake a long road of progression in which faithfulness is rewarded and honesty prevails. Enjoy the journey.

Technical Terms

Counter-clockwise

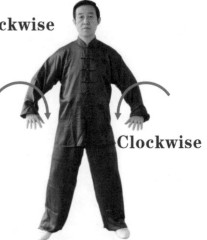

Rotate Clockwise: is defined as the turning movement towards the right side of the body in a circle or twining motion when you look at your arm rotate from your own eyes position. It is shown on the diagram with arrow and line of dots.

Clockwise

Rotate Counter Clockwise: is defined as the turning movement towards the left side of the body in a circle or twining motion when you look at your arm rotate from your own eyes position. It is shown on the diagram with arrow and solid line.

Hook: The fingers are bunched together with the crook of the wrist relaxed do not bend too much and form a rigid curve. Over bending of the wrist can cause tension on your arm and shoulders. Keeping the wrist in a leader position to direct the strength and internal energy flow.

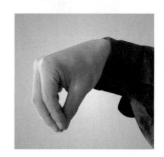

Fist: The fingers are clenched together with the thumb folded over the index and middle fingers as shown in the diagram. Keep fingers relaxed and loosely hold the fist during the movement and only tighten your fist at the last moment of energy releasing. Keep the fist straight forward from your forearm.

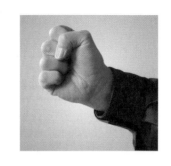

Palm: Chen Style Taijiquan requires the palm to be like a row of roof titles. The thumb and the little finger are intending to push toward each other slightly from distance, while the index, middle and ring finger all stay straight naturally and stretch out slightly to the rear. All five fingers are slightly bunched together, but without using any stiff strength (no tension). The centre of the palm is empty and the middle finger is the key finger of your intention during Tai Chi practice.

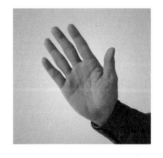

Empty step: Place the ball of the foot on the floor with toes touching the floor lightly and no weight or only very limited weight (10%) on the toes. Most of your weight is placed on the supporting leg.

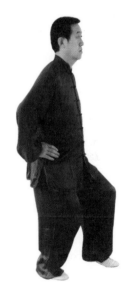

Weight: Weight is defined as your centre of gravity. In Chen Style Tai Chi the weight normally is deployed on both legs by percentage. either 40% and 60% or 30 and 70%. So, in the book when we indicate where the weight is, it means that approx. 60-70% of the weight is placed on that leg unless we say whole weight or specify exactly the percentage of the weight.

Tai Chi Chuan – Taijiquan: Taijiquan is the Mandarin spelling and Tai Chi Chuan is the Cantonese spelling and it means Tai Chi martial arts or Kung Fu under the guidance of Tai Chi philosophy.

Tai Chi – Taiji: Tai Chi and Taiji in terms are the same thing. Taiji is the Mandarin spelling and Tai Chi is the Cantonese spelling and it is an ancient Chinese philosophy - Yin and Yang.

Tai Chi stance: This is posture to stand still with both arms holding in a circle in front of your chest and fingures toward each other. Thumb pointing upward slightly and separate from others fingures. Weight is placed in the centre between two feet and both feet separate shoulder-width wide with both toes pointing outward slightly. bend both knees slightly and relax the hips. Head erect and body upright. Keep chin in and sink the chest down slightly. The crown of your head lifts up slightly as if you are holding a cup of coffee on top of your head lightly. Tongue touches the upper pallet with eyes lightly closed or looking forward downward. Breath in and out using your nose and let the breath deeply going through to your lower abdomen (Dantian). This is the best posture to feel the Tai Chi energy flow inside of your body. Once you have experienced the nice feeling of internal energy inside your body, it is recommended that you extend this feeling into all the movements when you practice the forms.

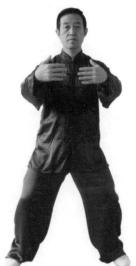

Bow Step: In traditional Chinese Martial Arts the Bow Step has a bent front leg and straight back leg with both feet firmly on the floor. In Tai Chi this move has a softening in the back knee and outward turn of the knee producing a more relaxed and flexible stance.

Silk Reeling Energy: This is a set of turning and spiraling movements which improve body stretching and flexibility removing blockages along the acupuncture channel maintaining good flow of internal energy. This feature differentiates Chen Style Tai Chi from the other styles of Tai Chi. It includes single hand and double hand movements working in co-operation with the feet .

Dantian: It is an acupuncture point located just three fingers width lower than your navel. It is considered the centre store of internal energy and focus point of the breath during Tai Chi practice. This is the most sensitive area where you can feel the increasing of Qi energy.

Baihui: An acupuncture point located on the top of the head connecting internal energy with sky energy. In Tai Chi, Baihui is considered the important point for internal energy flow and spiritual activities. It is considered the leader or commander of the whole body and energy.

Yongquan: Is an acupuncture point located at the centre of the sole of the foot (the place that does not touch the floor). It is a connecting point between your body and the earth.

Acknowledgments

The original book was written by Grandmaster Chen Zhenglei, translated by Xu Hailiang and published by Zhongzhou Publishing House in Zhengzhou city, Henan Province, P. R. China in September 2002. It is published in both Chinese and English and is entitled 'The Chen Style Taijiquan for life Enhancement' with ISBN: 7-5348-2181-9.

The content of the book in Chinese is of excellent quality and invaluable for those people who are interested in learning Chen Style Taijiquan. Unfortunately, the English translation of the book does not convey all the original correct meanings of the Chinese.

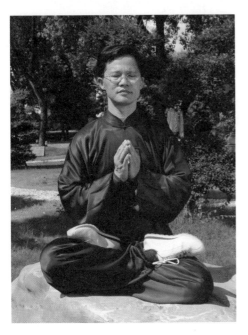

When I saw this book for the first time I was very excited about it as I thought that my students would have an English version of the Chen Style Taijiquan technique book to read. However after I read through this book, I became concerned about the clarity of the English translation of the book, particularly when I received feed back from those students who had read it. Many sentences in the book either lost their original meanings or offered only a very poor English translation. After discussion with Grandmaster Chen Zhenglei, I therefore decided to retranslate the book from its original Chinese content completely with clear and concise English.

As this newly translated book is in English and is to be distributed in English speaking countries in the West, I broadened the content of the book adding new chapters with answers for the most common questions that come from Taijiquan practitioners in the West. It includes the benefits, experience and knowledge that Western practitioners have gained from Taijiquan. There is a series of interviews with individual Taijiquan practitioners around the UK by journalist, Tim Birch. There are also dialogues with myself, Master Liming Yue, interviewed by Danny Chisholm, Nick Taylor and Anthony Rushton.

In order to make my English translation accurate and easy to understand while still capturing and communicating the original meaning of the Chinese version of the book, I have worked very closely with a group of my senior students who are currently working as Chen Style Taijiquan instructors in the UK. First I wrote a literal English translation of the Chinese. Then my students would

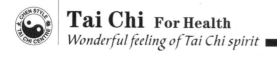

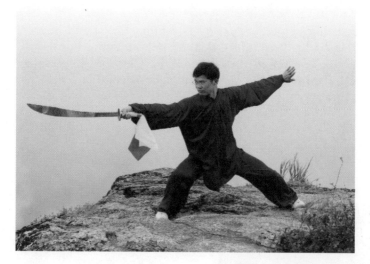

explain the meaning of the sentence to me from their own understanding. At the same time I also explained the original meaning of the Chinese to my students. We would not put any sentence into the book until both myself and my senior students compared the meanings carefully and we were all fully satisfied that the translation of the sentence matched with the Chinese meaning. Our goal was to publish a high quality English version of Chen Style Taijiquan which lets all the practitioners in the world receive the maximum benefits of the style.

To improve the quality of this book, I chose to use high resolution imagery and print in full colour. A further development is the addition of an instructional DVD for absolute clarity and convenience in the study and practice of Taijiquan. During the period of writing the book many of my senior students and friends have given me a lot of help. In particular, while I was translating the instructional chapter of the 18 Short Form, Ploutarchos (Pluto) Vlachopoulos, Sue Johnson and John Bolwell helped me as a team. After I finished the translation of the form movements from Chinese, we used one person to read the instruction of the form while others tried to follow the instructions to demonstrate the movements as described in the book. At all times 1 ensured everything went correctly. This process ensured that all the translation in the book is accurate and understandable to all readers.

After I drew up the first draft I sent it around to a group of my senior students and other friends to proof read and asked them to give me feed back. Those people include: Peter Donaldson, Bill Wilkinson, Geoff Leversedge, Dan Chisholm, Nick Taylor, Linda Wilkinson, Steven Burton, Anthony Rushton, Tim Birch, and Shabir Akhtar. I also remember that one day I took a copy of a draft to one of my classes at Age Concern, Ashton-under-Lyne, Greater Manchester. Students in the class separated the entire book into sections and took home one set each to read through and bring back with their feedback at following classes. There are many stories like this and I am very appreciative of all the kind help

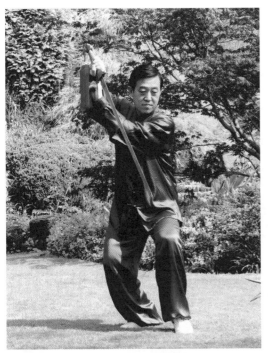

from all of those people. In addition I would like to mention my senior students in Manchester including: Cemil Egeli, Bruce Li and Gillian Egeli for their support and dedication over the years. This also includes those people who have given help in any format but whom are not named in the book.

It has taken me two and a half year of hard work, and now the final draft of the book has been settled. I hope every reader enjoys it and gains great benefits from the book.

Master Liming Yue, 8th August 2005

Sword Posture – Closing the Door.

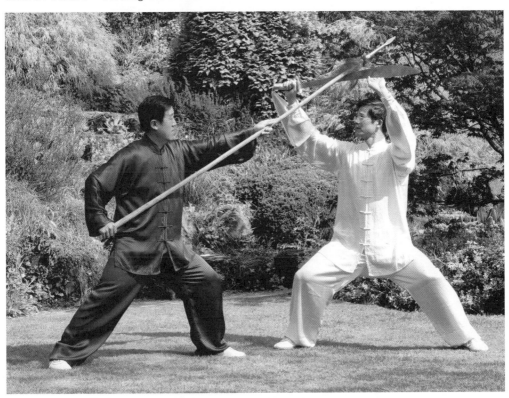

Sabre aganst Spear, demonstrated by Grandmaster Chen Zhenglei and Master Liming Yue in Manchester, UK 2003.

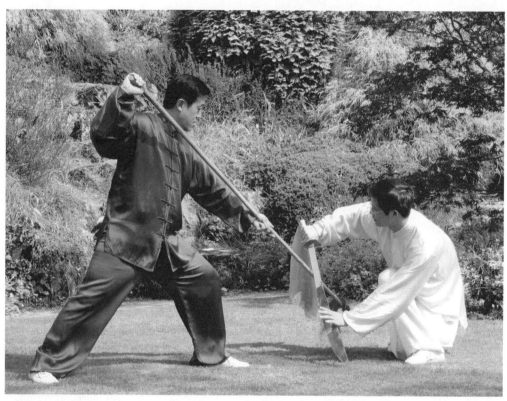

Sabre defends the attack of the Spear.

成功源自貴人相助

Introduction to Chen Style Taijiquan
Written by Master Liming Yue

Chen Style Tai Chi (Taijiquan) was created in Chenjiagou Village, Wenxian County, Henan Province, China in the late Ming Dynasty, almost 400 years ago, by the 9th generation Chen family member, General Chen Wangtin. Following a decorated military career, General Chen retired to Chenjiagou where he began formulating an internal martial art that incorporated the wisdom of the ancient philosophy of Yin and Yang, with specialized breathing techniques, and a profound understanding of the internal energy meridians "jingluo" used in Traditional Chinese Medicine.

Such was its intrinsic power that the art was only passed from master to student in great secrecy and remained hidden for almost 300 years. It was not until the 14th generation of the Chen family (around 120 years ago) that Grandmaster Chen Changxing taught the art to Yang Luchan, a household servant. Yang Luchan (founder of Yang Style Tai Chi) was the first to take the art away from the village and quickly his reputation spread throughout China as an unbeatable master using this fascinating martial art.

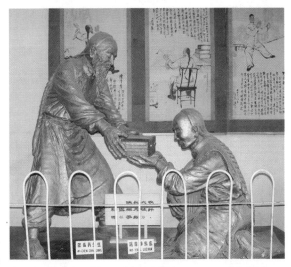

Grandmaster Chen Changxing passes his Tai Chi books to Yang Luchan (the founder of Yang Style Tai Chi)

During the rapid popularization of Yang Style Tai Chi, the Chen Family Style remained within Chenjiagou, the village members being dedicated to the advancement and preservation of all aspects of the tradition, just as their ancestors had done for almost 400 years.

Chen Style Tai Chi has recently made its appearance on the international scene and is fast becoming the most popular form of Tai Chi in the world today. Old and new students alike are beginning to appreciate why generations of the Chen family were determined to maintain their sacred art in its purest form, so that everyone may experience the maximum benefits under their guidance.

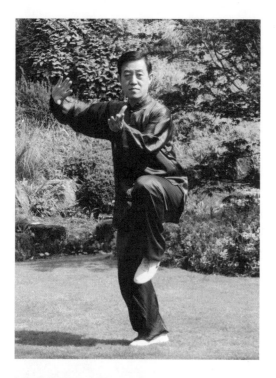

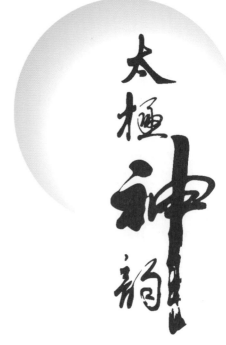

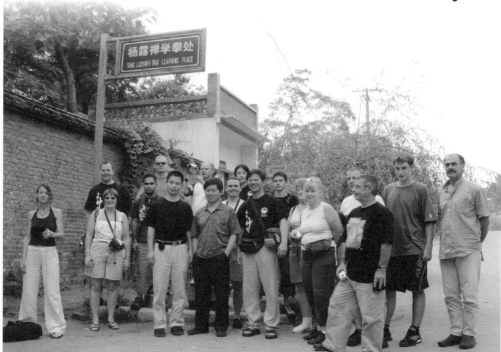

Group Picture in front of the house where Yang Luchan (The founder of Yang Style Tai Chi) learnt Chen Style Tai Chi in the Chenjiagou Village, Wen County, Henan Province, P. R. China 2004.

Chapter One
The Principles of Chen Style Tai Chi for Health

Chen Style Tai Chi for Health presents the most valuable and essential health aspects of Chen Style Taijiquan which include unique methods for increasing internal energy, energy collection and energy control. The exercises also help vitalize and enhance mental capacity. In combining the body movements of Taijiquan with the movement of the breath it is also possible to develop and improve spiritual awareness.

The exercises or body movements that will be discussed in this book, are the Foundation exercises (warm up, footstep exercises and silk reeling exercises), Qigong exercises (meditation, Tai Chi stance and energy collection) and the Chen Style 18 Short Form, which together, form the principles of Chen Style Taijiquan for Health.

All of these exercises are easy and straightforward for people to learn and practice. They are very effective in helping to reduce high blood pressure, heart disease, arthritis, neurasthenia, gastric ulcers and other chronic diseases. These exercises can also benefit weight loss, stress relief, disruptive sleep patterns, and greatly enhance health and fitness.

The practice of Taijiquan does not require a big space or any special equipment for personal training. It can be practiced at any time of day or night, indoors or out. Taijiquan is suitable for all people, regardless of age, sex, or level of fitness.

太極天天走　治病又強身

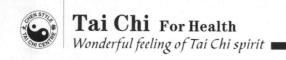

Section One
The Features of the Exercises

Tai Chi for Health contains still exercises, meditation and the Tai Chi stance, alone with dynamic moving exercises called forms. It places equal emphasis on external body movements and internal energy control. Mental awareness is combined with body movements. The conscious mind focuses on the movements, directing the body to move through the forms.

During practice, keep quiet, calm and relaxed. Follow the principle "When one part of the body moves, the whole body moves accordingly. When one part of the body is motionless, the whole body is still". Let awareness, body movements and breathing combine to complement each other, co-operating and working together simultaneously. Your body and the space around you should form one unit. Collect all of the sky and earth energy (Qi) into the body and use it to nourish and replenish yourself. At the same time release harmful negative energy from the body. This helps to achieve good health and a long and happy life.

After a period of practice, your Qi energy, inherited at birth, will start to concentrate in your Dantian (located three fingers width below the navel) and energy surges throughout the body. As energy increases, feelings become stronger and your mood improves, making you happier, more cordial and more tolerant of other people, eliminating nervousness and anxiety. Strengthening Qi energy in this way is very beneficial for health, boosting the immune system and helping to protect against sickness and disease.

Once in command of energizing the body, the next step is to learn how to release energy. Releasing energy forms the powerful opening or closing elements of self- defense. Great care needs to be taken when using the energy release movements contained within the form. Energy release can both protect you from injury and also cause injury to an opponent.

In general, Tai Chi movements are very flexible and fluid. For practice purposes, you should follow the principles above and try to be as natural as possible. Try to avoid focusing purely on the movements themselves. Also try to remain aware of the philosophy behind the movements and your own internal feeling of energy.

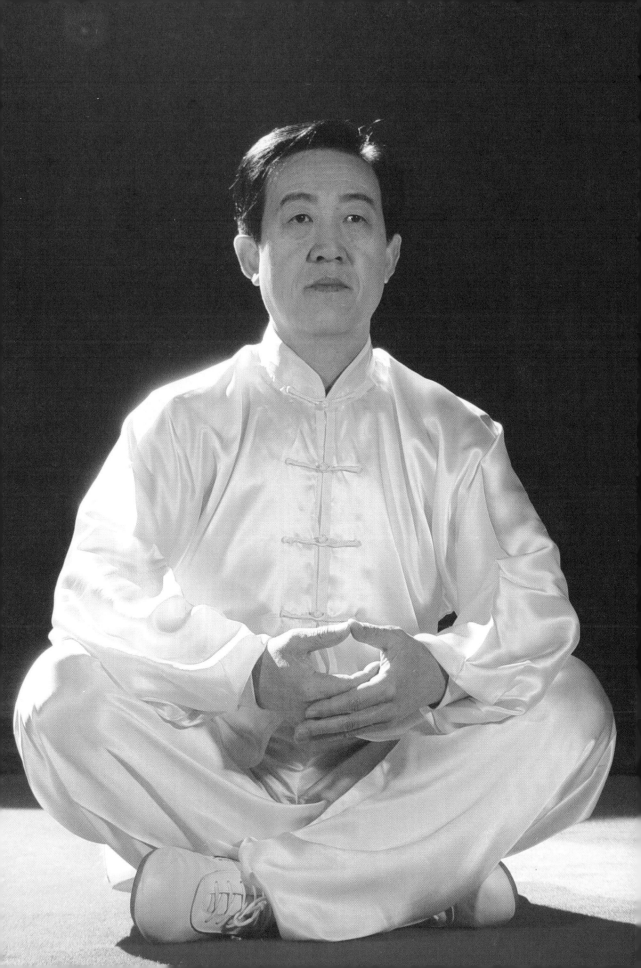

Section Two
The Health Benefits of the Exercises

1. Enhancing the health of the nervous system and conditioning the reflex reactions.

All of the bodily functions in your daily life are guided by the nervous system. In particular, the co-ordination of the body muscles and the regulation and control of the internal organs. Most Taijiquan exercises require a focused and relaxed mind during practice. As a result of this, the exercises stimulate and enhance the energy flow within the body, which in

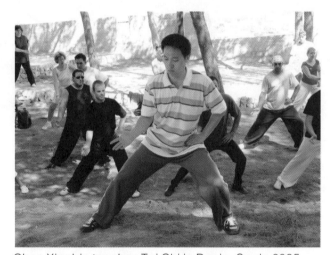

Chen Xiaobin teaches Tai Chi in Denia, Spain 2005

turn reinforces the ability of the nervous system to concentrate and focus more easily. In addition, as the nervous system improves, the peripheral nervous system is enhanced, as is your sensitivity within sensory organs such as the eyes, ears, nose, tongue, skin etc. This makes your reflexes and reactions noticeably faster, and can also help to improve your ability in learning new skills. Regular practitioners of Taijiquan find that they feel more energized and fresh, thinking more clearly and feeling happier, with a better and more efficient motivation for work.

Normally, people's emotions are highly linked to the state of their health. Positive motivation and healthy ambition are important factors for good health. An excess of the emotions such as happiness, anger, worry, thinking, sadness, paranoia or depression and fear can cause health problems which can often appear as physical symptoms of illness. In China, these are called the seven emotions. According to ancient Chinese medical philosophy the seven emotions are considered as the root cause of illness. They are connected to the six internal organs of the human body. If you are too happy, it can cause heart problems. However if you are too angry, it can cause liver problems. Too much worry and thinking can cause spleen problems while too much sorrow can cause lung problems. Excess paranoia or depression can cause kidney damage and excessive fear can damage your gallbladder. There are also six external physical conditions that can contribute to sickness, they include excesses of wind, cold, heat, dampness, dryness and fire. Normally, the six external causes are not strong enough to create illness, but when one or more of the seven emotions are out of balance, the body's defence is weakened against the six external influences entering the body and causing illness. This is why the ancient Chinese medical book Neijing places emphasis on keeping quiet and ignoring any external interruptions, clearing your mind and focusing on your internal feeling when you are practicing Qigong, which is also a key requirement for Taijiquan.

Stressful, busy, fast and intensive modern city life causes people many problems such as stress, short temper, anxiety, inefficiency and poor sleep patterns. Tai Chi for Health exercises utilize the Neijing principle of using your own mind to relax your body and spirit, relieve stress, and calm the seven emotions. This reduces the chances of becoming ill, and improves overall health.

2. Improving the condition of bones, joints and muscles and the ability to exercise

Tai Chi for Health exercises are based on turning, spiraling and twisting movements. These types of movement co-ordinate the bones, joints and muscles, increasing the density, thickness and strength of the bones, the muscles also becoming

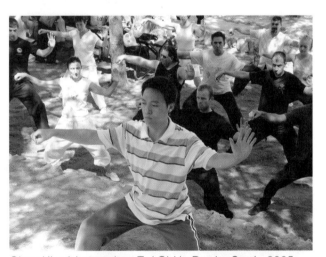

Chen Xiaobin teaches Tai Chi in Denia, Spain 2005

stronger. In turn, this makes bones harder and more resistant to being injured or broken. The joints and the tendons around them also become more flexible and elastic. This is good for the well-being of the joints and muscles, improving the practice of Taijiquan and significantly increasing your ability to apply or defeat a lock movement. Beyond that, the sensitivity gained from practicing these exercises improves both the relaxation of mind and body as well as enhancing the ability to react to external stimuli.

All of these twisting and spiraling movements are controlled by the mind, based on the relaxation of the body. The whole body co-operates with itself, with muscle fibre becoming longer (because of the twisting movements), more elastic and stronger. One of the benefits of this kind of exercise is its ability to reduce the amount of fat around the muscles and open the pores

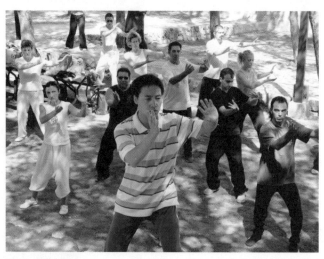

Chen Xiaobin teaches Tai Chi in Denia, Spain 2005

of your skin, resulting in the skin looking and feeling smoother, softer and healthier. A further benefit is that slim people are able to put more muscle on, and over-weight people are able to get rid of excess fat, aiding weight loss.

3. Strengthening the digestive system and improving the respiratory functions

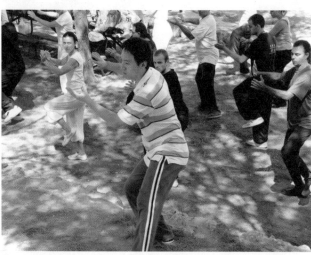

Chen Xiaobin teaches Tai Chi in Denia, Spain 2005

The basic functions of the digestive system are to ingest food, absorb nutrients and expel waste. In Chinese medicine the digestive system and a person's state of health is closely connected to the ability of the six internal organs to function correctly. Tai Chi for Health exercises are smooth, gentle and slow. The breath naturally follows the body movements which, in turn, allows internal energy to circulate more freely inside the body, flowing through all of the internal organs. The muscles of the abdominal region benefit functions of the digestive system greatly from long and deep breaths taken

During Tai Chi exercise. It feels like a soft massage on the stomach and the intestines. Whilst exercising in this way secretions from the digestive glands increase, reducing digestion times and improving the absorption and assimilation of the nutrition of food. Thus practicing Tai Chi for Health exercises improves appetite, enhances the helps to cure dyspepsia, gastrointestinal neurosis, gastric ulcers, anorexia, bilimbi and eating disorders.

Tai Chi for Health exercises require the body movements and breath to co-operate with each other, allowing Qi energy to flow to the four extremities (the tips of fingers and toes), resulting in the breath becoming slower, deeper and longer. During such a process, the contraction and expansion of the abdominal muscles can be improved, and the traction force between the thoraxes increased. The contact area between capillary vessels and alveoli enlarges, improving lung capacity and efficiency. A benefit of this is being able to maintain your concentration longer without getting tired and improving your working efficiency.

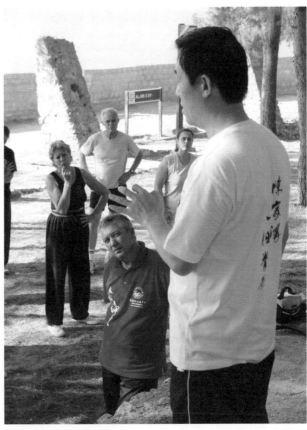
Grandmaster Chen Zhenglei in Denia, Spain 2005

4.Strengthening the functions of the heart, improving the condition of the blood vessels

Taijiquan life enhancement exercises can make the cardiac muscle fibre wider and stronger, the wall of the heart thicker, the contracting ability better and blood circulation easier. In addition, it can improve the flexibility and fortitude of the arterial wall, making the diameter of coronary arteries wider. These changes improve the functioning of the blood vessel system which, in turn helps nutrition to be absorbed by the digestive organs, improves oxygen absorption into the lungs and assists the secretion of hormones by internal glands to organs and tissues. Regular practice of Taijiquan can greatly help in improving all of the functions of the heart. The heart rate when you are quiet is lower than usual, slightly increasing when you are moving normally, and greatly increasing when exercising vigorously, but resuming its slow rate faster than usual. Overall, Taijiquan is beneficial to homeostasis, metabolism and the stability of the internal organs.

5. Stimulating the internal energy, smoothing the Jingluo

Jingluo (acupuncture meridians, or channels) are the main blood and Qi energy channels and are directly related to the body and mind's state of health. If the channels are free of blockages health will be good. If the channels are blocked sickness can occur. That is why according to ancient Chinese medical philosopher, Lingshu- Jingbi says "those 12 channels are the source of people's living, as well as people's sickness. To find out and cure the sickness you have to check the 12 channels and their condition." Essentially, Traditional Chinese Medicine (TCM) is a lifetime of continuously studying the 12 channels.

Maintaining the channels by keeping them unblocked helps to prevent illness and maintains the body's natural balance and harmony.

Taijiquan and Qigong exercises have many different methods of practice. Whichever method you choose, the final goal and fundamental Purpose is to increase the level of Qi energy within the body and drive it through the 12 main channels, producing a half-body energy circle (Xiaozhoutian) or a full-body energy circle (Dazhoutian). The benefits of this can vary from the prevention of sickness to maintaining a good level of fitness, helping to keep the mind sharp and keen while enjoying a long and healthy life.

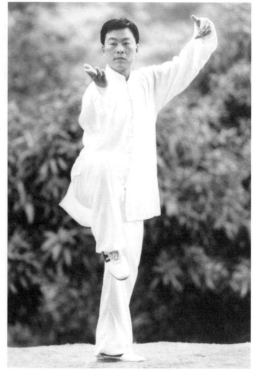

Senior instructor Zhang Dongwu in the Chenjiagou Tai Chi Centre China

Internal energy (Qi) is the vital living force existing within every human body. The flow of internal energy is integral to the health of the individual. This internal energy is present from birth but how it develops and strengthens depends upon the level of practice and training that is undertaken by each individual. As long as you practice with a reasonable method, the internal energy will begin to increase in power and become a united force within the body. The outcome being that one can use this enhanced energy for self-defence, maintaining a healthy life, enhancing the ability to rid oneself of sickness and preventing diseases from entering the body in the first place.

The Tai Chi for Health life enhancement method of exercising requires a relaxed body, a calm mind and a quiet environment. Using the mind in combination with correct body posture and movements to direct internal energy increases Qi circulation within the body. Once the internal energy starts to get more powerful, Qi energy will flow with greater ease through the 12 main energy channels and spread throughout the whole body. Under your control and direction, the internal energy moves through your heart, maintaining it in a good state by relaxing it and making it more flexible, thus helping to prevent heart attacks. If moved through the kidneys, the internal energy makes them stronger, making you feel

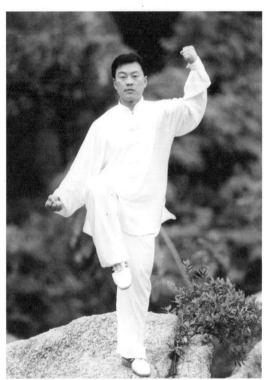

Senior instructor Zhang Dongwu in the Chenjiagou Tai Chi Centre China

more energized and revitalized. When the energy moves through the lungs it makes your breathing much longer and deeper, moving oxygen to the brain more efficiently. Also, because the breathing goes up and down to your Dantian (lower abdomen), it results in shortening the length of time in which you are out of breath after exercising or undertaking strenuous activity. Once the energy passes through the liver it helps to cool it down, relieving it from any 'anger-heat'. Then, if it is directed through the spleen, it improves its ability to work with the stomach which, in turn, helps the digestive system as well as the absorption of nutrition. Direct the energy up to the head and it brings a calmer and more refreshed feeling. As the blood supply increases and the brain gets more oxygen, the optical nerves relax, making your eyesight sharper. It also the arteries, therefore helping to prevent heart attacks. When it travels through your hair, it makes the hair very sensitive, and the scalp more efficient in getting rid of all the waste fluids when you perspire. An ancient Chinese medical health expert once said, "use your mind to direct your Qi energy according to your own body's requirements and, in this way, rid the body of any sickness. Many of the internal sicknesses can thus be cured."

Section Three
The Key Requirements and Main Details for Exercising

1. Being relaxed, calm and natural

Relax your whole body. Relax the internal organs, bone structure, muscles, skin, and hair. Nothing should be tense whilst practicing.

Calm the mind. Make your spirit clear, calm yourself down, get rid of any unnecessary thoughts and concentrate on your practice. Breathe naturally. While you practice, do not hold your breath and do not use stiff strength. In the beginning allow your body movements to co-operate with your breathing naturally. Do not force your breathing to go along with your body movements whilst you are a beginner.

2. Co–ordinating the mind and Qi together, uniting the body with the spirit

Use the mind to direct your Qi and make your movements work in conjunction with your breathing. When your mind is concentrated on a movement, your Qi energy follows and then your strength comes. All in order, but all as one. The principle of co-ordinating the breathing with the movements is "when the movement is closing, breathe in and whilst opening, breathe out. When the movement is pulling in, breathe in, and when the movement is pushing out, breathe out. When the movement is rising up, breathe in and when the movement is dropping down, breathe out. When you collect the energy, breathe in and when you release energy or strike, breathe out". In general, everything has to be natural. Do not force your breathing to make it long and deep in the early stages. It will make correct breathing harder not easier. It also clogs energy and clarity of thought, hampering training. Keeping it natural and taking it easy are highly recommended training methods.

3. Keep the body upright and centralized. Distinguish between Solidity and Emptiness

Whatever form your practice takes, Taijiquan, Moving Qigong or Still Qigong, the body should always be upright and centered. As a general rule, you should not lean to any side and you should not move your upper body around without this being a requirement of the whole movement. As a special requirement, keep your head erect and relax your neck and shoulders. Drop your elbows down, keep your chest in and relaxed, sink your waist down and relax the hips. When you move or rotate the body, your head, along with your central body and the four limbs should all be co-ordinated. Eyes should look forward in a level direction, not up or down. The acupuncture points Baihui (top of the head) and Changqiang (between the tip of the coccyx and anus) should be linked together and synchronized with each other.

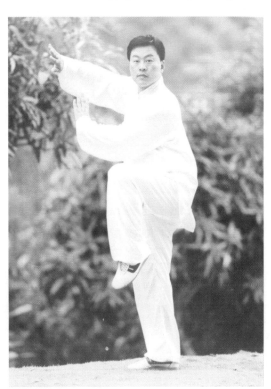

Whilst practicing, pay attention to the transference of weight. Distinguish between Yin (emptiness) and Yang (solidity). Make sure your internal energy is flowing, and the structural strength of the posture is correct, using natural and flowing movements. If any of the above requirements are not met, you should consider adjusting your movements during your training.

Senior instructor Zhang Dongwu in the Chenjiagou Tai Chi Centre China

Whilst you practice, you have to follow the golden rule, which is, 'one moves, all move'. When your hand moves, the rest of your body follows. Pay attention to the whole body, make sure that hands, eyes, body movements and feet integrate and co-operate together. Place emphasis on moving your internal energy, spirit, strength and energy release in the same direction. Always follow these principles when you practice.

4. Length of Practice

The practicing time can vary between 20 minutes to one hour for beginners, gradually increasing. The amount of exercise one should take depends on the individual level of fitness. For a healthy person, after you practice your body should feel a little bit tired. This will vary according to each person's level of fitness, but one should pay attention not to overdo it. Your mind and spirit should feel revitalized. For less fit people, the practice time should be shorter and less intensive with higher postures. The practice time and intensity of practice should be increased and the postures lowered gradually over time as your level of fitness increases.

Ill people should not become overtired during practice. Once you feel tired stop exercising and rest until you feel fit enough to continue your practice. It is recommended to have short breaks in the middle of a training session. Seriously ill people should consult their health consultant or G.P. (Medical Doctor) and discuss the health conditions with the class instructor before taking on any Tai Chi exercise.

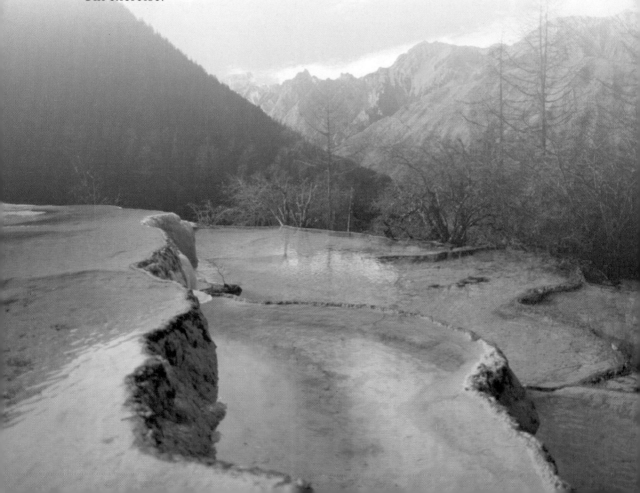

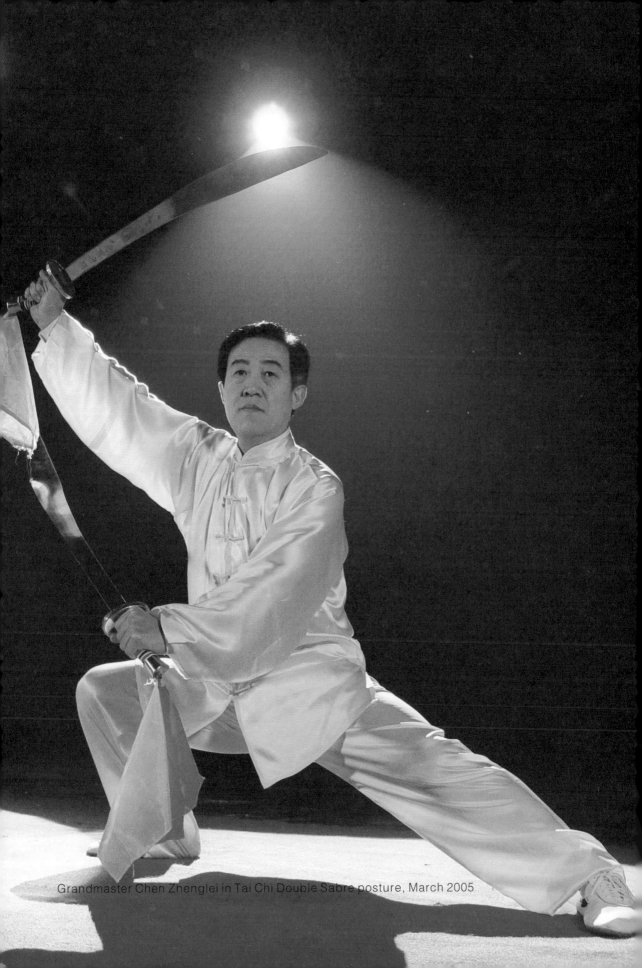

Grandmaster Chen Zhenglei in Tai Chi Double Sabre posture, March 2005

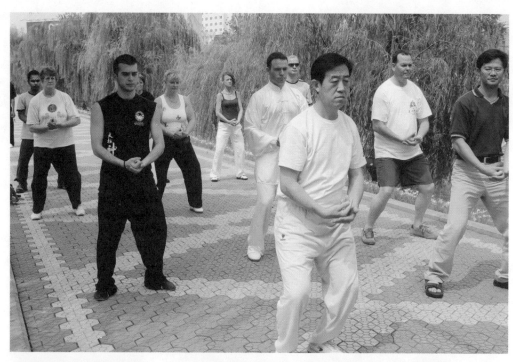

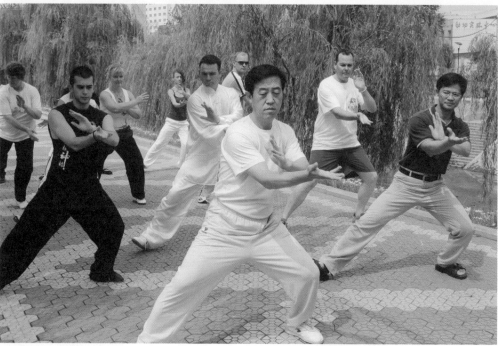

Morning practice in the park in China during the China Trip 2004 organized by Chen Style Tai Chi Centre UK. Training lead by Grandmaster Chen Zhenglei.

Chapter Two
The Foundation Training Exercises
Section One
Warm up exercises

Blood is described as being in the state of Yin, and Qi energy is in the state of Yang. Blood is the source of Qi energy, and Qi energy helps the blood to flow and circulate in a symbiotic relationship.

The Warm Up exercises consist of rolling, stretching and loosening the fingers, wrists, elbows, shoulders, chest, waist, hips, knees, ankles and toes. This relaxes the muscles and tendons, along with a stretching and loosening of the joints. The Warm Up exercises also helps the blood to circulate more efficiently. This in turn makes the Qi energy stronger, helping the blood to circulate even more efficiently and so on.

The Warm Up exercises are preparation exercises prior to practicing Chen Style Taijiquan. They are also excellent as a warm up exercise for other sporting activities as well.

These exercises can also be extremely beneficial when practiced purely in their own right, as well as a warm up to more strenuous activity. They are good for joints and tendons and can help to prevent arthritis. The exercises should be done until you begin to produce a mild sweat. This will ensure that the entire body is sufficiently warmed up, reducing the risk of strain or injury.

These exercises have been well received the world over and are suitable not only for Taiji practicioners but also for all types of people ranging from althletes to the elderly. These exercises are clearly demonstrated on the DVD.

[練拳不練功　到老一場空]

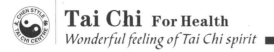

1 Circling head

Stand upright with your feet shoulder-width apart. Place both palms on both sides of the waist with the thumbs pointing backward and the fingers forward. Using your neck as the pivot, roll your head to the left, back, right, front and left again in a circular movement eight times. Do the same in the reverse direction. (Fig 2-1, 2-2, 2-3)

2-1

2-2

2-3

2 Wrist Rotating Exercise

Stand upright with your feet shoulder-width apart. Join your hands together in front of the body with the fingers interlaced. Rotate your wrists and in a circular motion in both directions, keeping your fingers, wrists, arms and shoulders relaxed. Repeat this movement 2x8 times. (Fig 2-4)

3 Arm Circling around Elbow exercise

Stand upright with your feet shoulder-Width apart. Hang both arms by your side at Waist level. (Fig 2-5) Move the arms (the movement should use the elbow as the pivot for your forearm movements as much as possible) in a circle. Your palms move inward, backward then move out to both sides of the body and finally reach the front of your body to form completed circular movements. (Fig 2-6) Repeat this movement many times (doing sets of 8 is preferable).

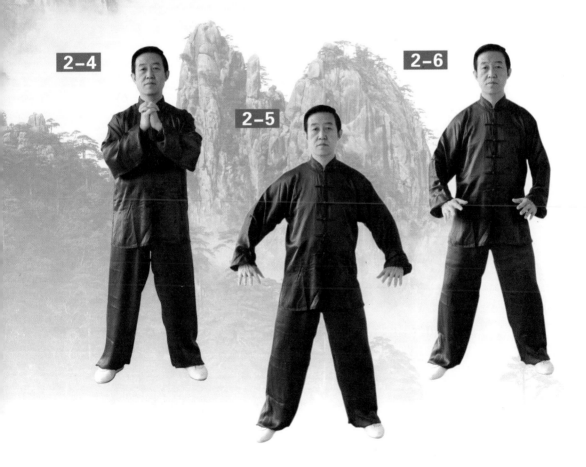

2-4

2-5

2-6

4 Elbow Circling around Shoulder

Stand upright with your feet shoulder width apart. Change both hands into hook-hands and place them on the front shoulders. Using both shoulder joints as pivots, start rotating the elbows in a circular movement. Both elbows move up, forward and then down in a circle. Do eight circles in both directions, repeating the exercise if necessary (2 sets of eight circles for e.g.) (Fig 2-7, 2-8, 2-9)

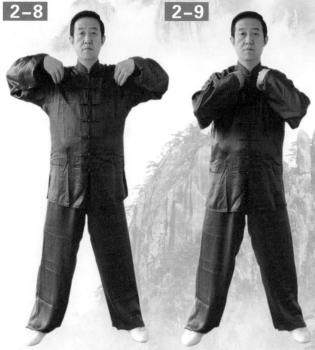

2-7

2-8

2-9

5 Chest-Stretching exercise

Stand upright with your feet shoulder width apart. Raise both arms horizontally in front of the chest with the palms facing down, elbows bent and fingers pointing toward each other. Move both elbows backwards and sideways twice so that the chest opens. (Fig 2-10) Then bring the forearms in front of your chest so that the right one is above the left one. This time move both arms back rotating them so that the palms face up and the whole arm is extended fully. After another two repetitions return to the starting position and repeat the first exercise with the elbows. Do both movements eight times. (Fig 2-11)

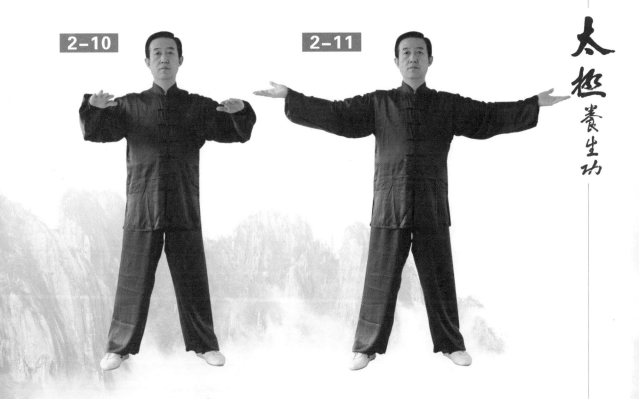

2-10 2-11

6 Arm Stretching exercise

Stand upright with your feet shoulder width apart and arms at your side. Raise the left hand up keeping the arm straight and the palm facing forward. Your right hand should be hanging by the right side of your body, palm facing back. Move both arms backward and forward four times simultaneously, (Fig 2-12) feeling your chest opening and expanding, and then swap the position of the arms, repeating the exercise for another four times. (Fig 2-13) Do two or three sets of this movement.

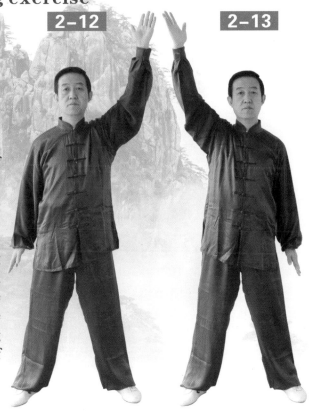

2-12 2-13

7 Arm Relax with Body Turning exercise

Stand upright with your feet shoulder-width apart and arms at the side. The shoulders, arms and hips should be relaxed and the knees slightly bent. Fix both feet on the floor and turn the body to the left and then to the right by using the waist. Following the movement of the body, swing both arms in the same direction. The hands should gently pat the body at the extremities of the movement. The arms should rise slowly so that the hands pat the body from the waist, until they are gently patting the body behind the shoulders. Eyes look to the rear-left of the body and the rear-right alternately, following the movement. (Fig 2-14, Fig 2-15) Repeat this exercises as many times as you like.

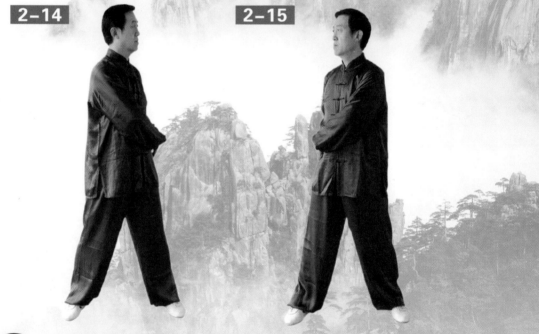

2-14 **2-15**

8 Waist Turning exercise

Stand upright with your feet shoulder-width apart. Clench both fists and raise them horizontally in front of the chest, bend the elbows and bring the fists to face each other. Keeping your feet still, twist your waist to one side roughly 45 degrees. Return to the starting position and do another twist (same direction) up to 90 degrees. (Fig 2-16) Do not over-twist! Do two twists in each direction (Fig 2-17), making the first a gentle one, and the second a harder one. Repeat this movement eight times in each direction.

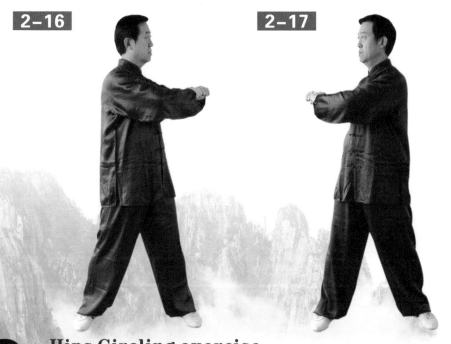

2-16   **2-17**

9 Hips Circling exercise

Stand upright with your feet shoulder-width apart. Place both hands on the sides of your waist with the thumbs pointing forward and the fingers pointing back. (Fig 2-18) Using the hips as a pivot, move them left, back, right and then forward in a circular motion, eight times. (Fig 2-19, 2-20) Change the direction of the movement and do another eight circles.

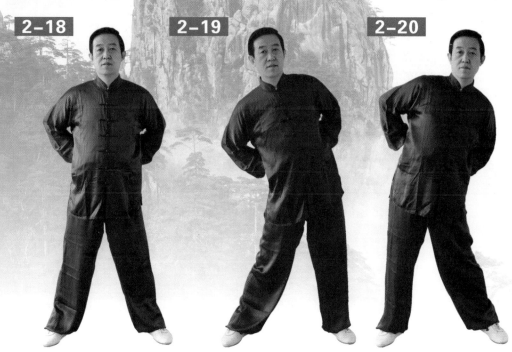

2-18   **2-19**   **2-20**

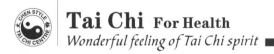
10 Knees Circling exercise

Stand upright with your feet shoulder width apart. Bend the knees and place both palms on the knees. Using the kneecaps as pivots rotate them in a circular motion, one clockwise and the other anticlockwise. (Fig 2-21) You can also place both feet together, the position of the palms unchanged, and using the knees as pivots rotate them from left to right for eight circles. (Fig 2-22) Repeat this movement on the opposite direction as well.

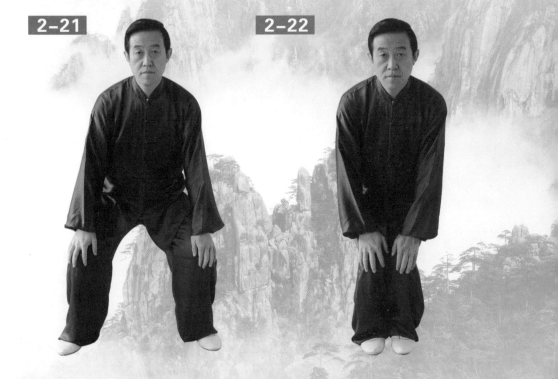

11 Ankles Rotating exercise

Stand upright with your feet slightly apart. Place hands on the sides of your waist, with your thumbs pointing backward, and your fingers forward. Shift the weight on to your right leg, the toes of the left foot just touching the floor. Using the toes of the left foot as a supporting point and the ankle joint as an axis, rotate the ankle in a circular motion. (Fig 2-23) Repeat the movement using the other leg. (Fig 2-24) Repeat this exercise as many times as you like.

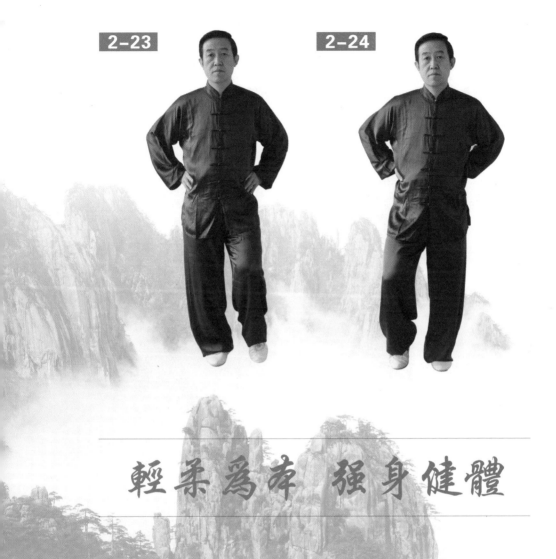

2-23

2-24

輕柔爲本　強身健體

12 Relaxing exercise

Stand upright with your feet slightly apart. Shift your weight onto the right leg and lift your left foot up whilst relaxing the hips and bending the knees. Move the arms back and turn your body to the right slightly. (Fig 2-25) Kick down with the left foot and at the same time throw both arms forward, relaxing the joints of the entire body. (Fig 2-26) Then shift your weight onto the left leg and repeat the movement. (Fig 2-27, 2-28) Repeat this exercise as many times as you like.

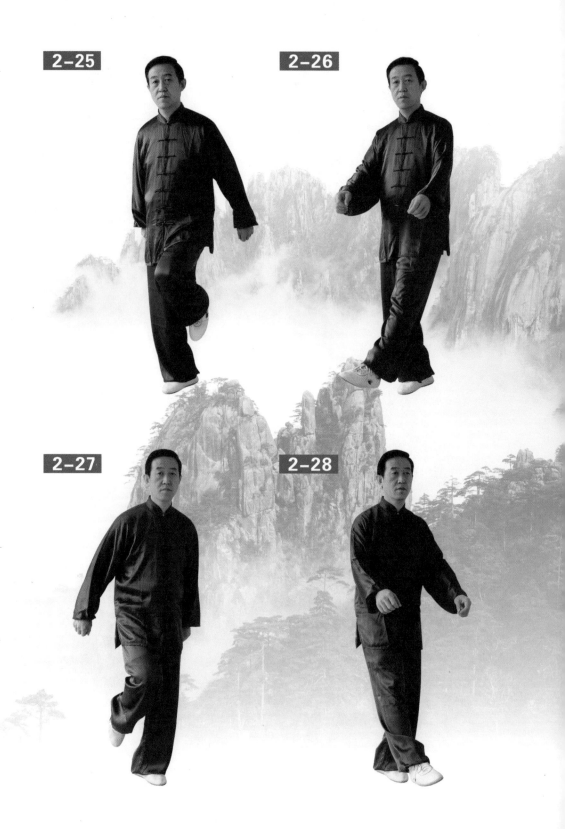

2-25

2-26

2-27

2-28

Section Two
Silk Reeling Energy Exercises

1.Single hand

1 Stand with your feet wide apart, knees bent, taking most (60-70%) of the weight on your left leg. Extend the left arm to the side at shoulder level with the palm facing forward. Place the right palm on the right side of the waist with the thumb pointing back and the fingers forward. Eyes look towards the left hand. (Fig 2-29)

2 Turn the body to the right slightly, moving the weight to the right leg. At the same time, move the left palm down and right rotating the arm counterclockwise, following the body movement in a semi circle in front of the abdomen. This is called - counter-clockwise arm rotating movement. (Fig. 2-30)

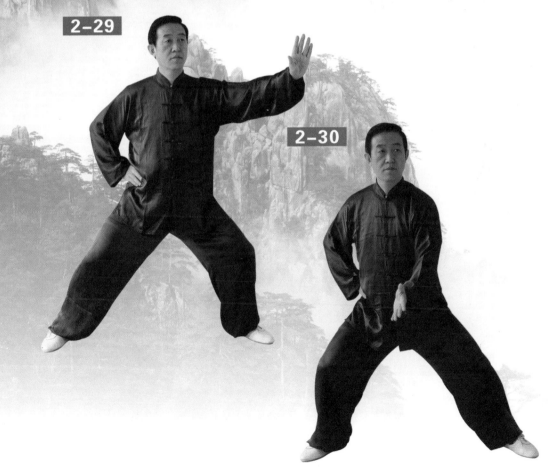

2-29

2-30

3 Continue to turn the body to the right. At the same time complete the semi circle in front of the chest with the palm turning to face out. The arm has to rotate clockwise This is called - clockwise arm rotating movement. Eyes look forward and right. (Fig 2-31)

4 Relax the left hip and turn the body to the left. Move the left palm up and left in an arc until it is above the left knee at shoulder level. Eyes look at the left palm. (Fig. 2-32)

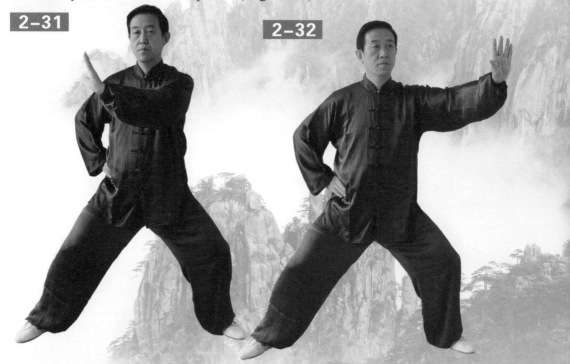

2-31

2-32

This single action will form a complete circle. Repeat this movement sixteen times or more (in sets of eight). Beginners must first understand the line of the movement, and then realize the movement of the weight, the turning of the waist and the changes of rotating the arms.

In this way, you will progress from being stiff and jerky to having smooth co-ordinated movements. When you have grasped the line of the movement well, incorporate your breathing into the movement. Inhale in the initial movement, collecting the fresh air (energy), from the centre of the palm, down to Dantian. Exhale in the final movement, where the internal energy flows from the Dantian to the fingers.

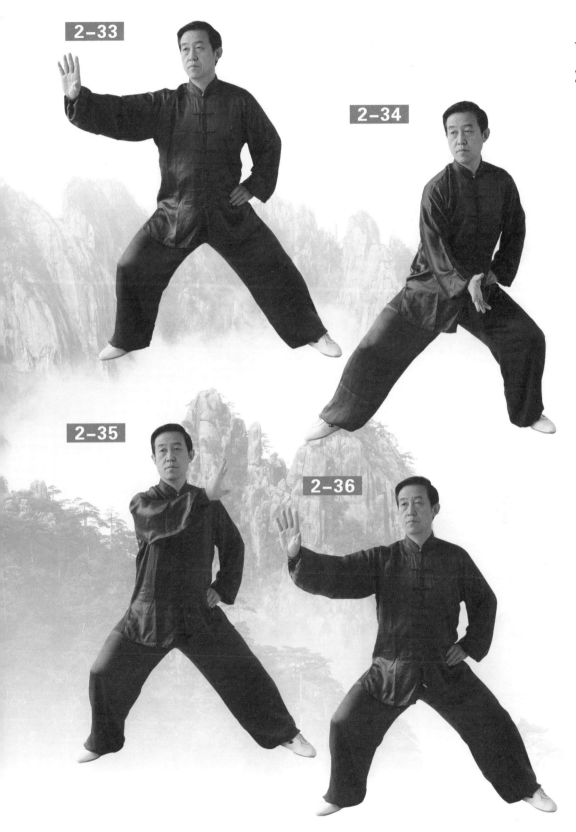

2-33

2-34

2-35

2-36

太極養生功

47

2. Both hands

1 From the Left Hand stance (Fig 2-32), turn the body slightly to the left, moving the right palm downward and leftward in a semi circle from the side of the waist in front of the abdomen (i.e. in a clockwise motion), warding off the left palm upward with a clockwise motion. Eyes look forward-right. (Fig 2-37)

2 Continue from the previous movement. Turn the body first to the left and then to the right with the weight moving to the right leg. At the same time, move the right palm leftward and upward, and then rightward and upward with counter clockwise rotating. Move the left palm downward and inward in front of the abdomen. Eyes look forward-left. (Fig 2-38) In this way, exercise the previous movements in a circular motion, so that the turning of the body and the rotation of both arms are co-ordinated.

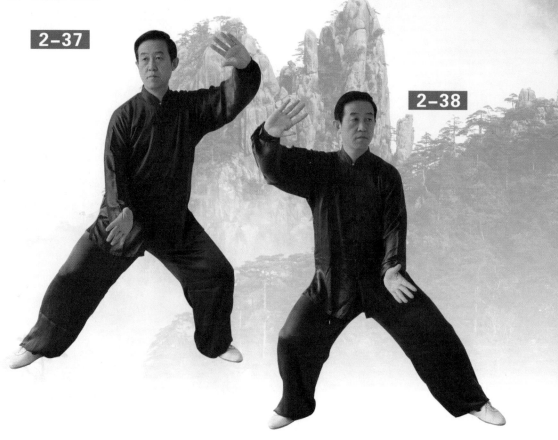

2-37

2-38

3. Wave the hand at the side of the body

1 Both legs form a left side bow step, with the weight mostly on the left leg. Left palm stretch out with elbow bent and keeping high as shoulder. The palm is vertically aligned above the left foot at shoulder height. Place the right palm on the right side of the waist, with the thumb pointing back and the rest of the fingers forward. Eyes look at the left palm. (Fig 2-39)

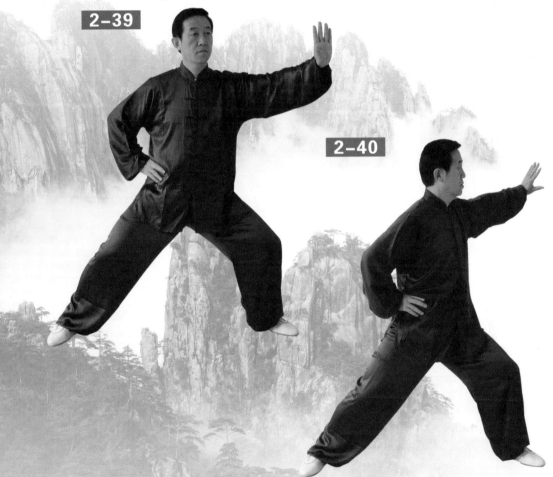

2-39

2-40

2 Continue from the previous movement. Turn the body to the left, move the left palm backward in an arc to the rear-left of the body. Eyes look at the left palm. (Fig 2-40)

3 Turn the body to the right and move the weight to the right leg. Move the left palm downward and forward above the left knee with arm rotate counter clockwise. Eyes look down and forward. (Fig 2-41)

4 Turn the body to the left slightly. Move the left palm upward with a counter clockwise arc movement whilst rotating the arm clockwise slightly until it is at shoulder level (Fig 2-42)

This movement consists of an opening and a closing that forms a circle. Complete this movement sixteen times or more, repeating the series for the right hand as well. The essential points of the exercise are the same as described already, simply reverse left and right. (Fig 2-43, 2-44, 2-45, 2-46)

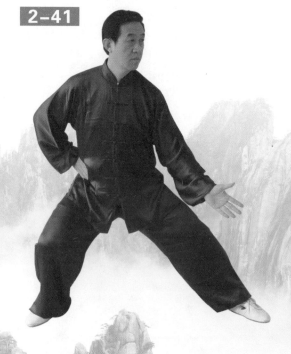

2-41

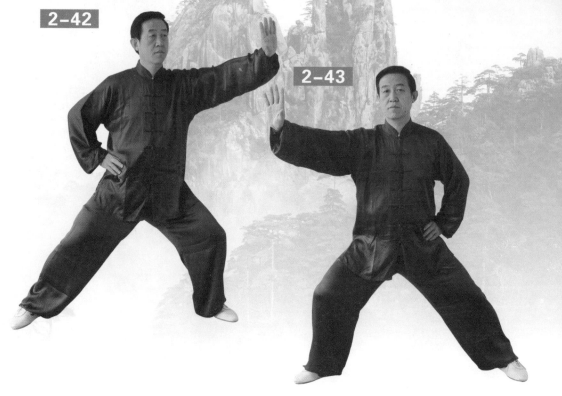

2-42

2-43

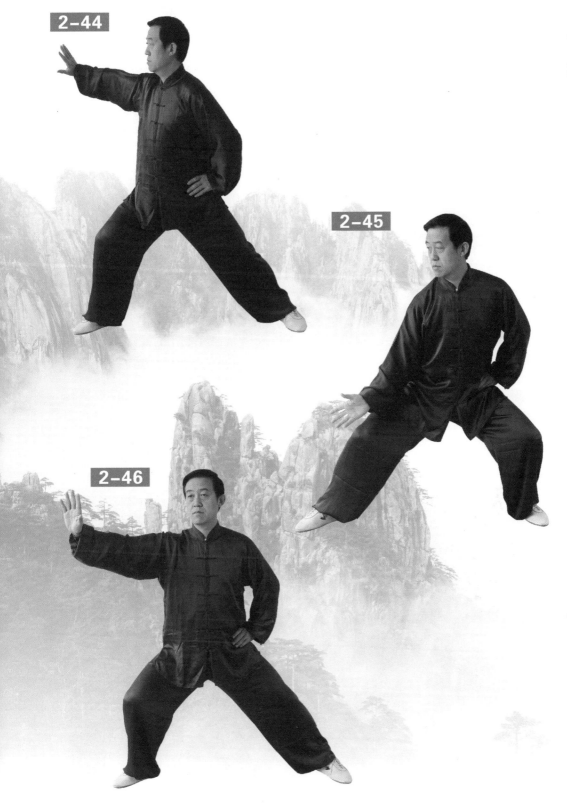

2-44

2-45

2-46

太極養生功

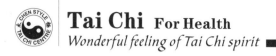

4. Deflect back on both sides of the body

1 Both legs form a right bow step. Place the left palm in front of the chest at shoulder level. Place the right palm on the right side of the waist. Eyes look forward. (Fig 2-47)

2 Continue from the previous movement. Turn the body to the left slightly and move the weight onto the left leg. At the same time, rotate the left palm clockwise whilst moving it down and back to the side of the waist with a counter clockwise movement. Rotate the right palm slightly clockwise whilst moving it back; raise it up and over in a circle then move it forward and right of the body, rotating it slightly counter clockwise. Eyes look forward. (Fig 2-48)

In this way, exercise the previous movements in a circular motion, paying attention to your waist, which serves as the main axis to initiate the movement of the arms. The waist initiates the shoulders, the shoulders initiate the elbows, and lastly the movement reaches the hands. When changing the direction of the palm from facing down to facing up and then rising, do not shrug the shoulders.

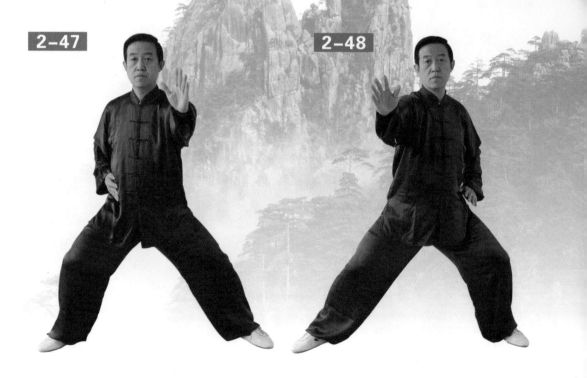

2-47

2-48

5. Twining both hands with forward step

1 Stand upright with the feet separate as shown on the diagram. Keep weight on the right leg and both palms pulling backward with finger pointing forward and palms facing outward. Eyes look forward. (Fig. 2-49)

2 Pulling both palms backward whilst the body turns to the right slightly. Eyes follow the palms movement. Keep weight on right leg and body sinks down slightly at your hips. (Fig. 2-50)

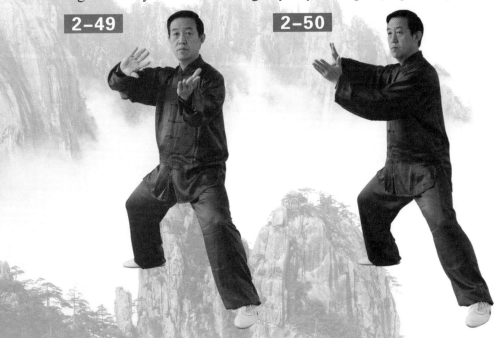

2-49

2-50

3 Turn body to the left whilst both palms move downward in an arc movements to the front of the abdomen with both arms rotating clockwise. Both palms face forward as shown on the diagram. Transfer the weight onto left leg during the movement. Eyes look forward. (Fig 2-51)

4 Rotate both arms counter clockwise and move both palms up then pulling/deflecting backward to its start position. Transfer weight back to right leg and turn body to the right as well. Eyes look forward. (Fig 2-52)Repeat the previous exercise for eight times then changing from left side to right. Pay attention to the waist, which serves as the main axis to initiate the movements of the arms, and use awareness to initiate the energy.

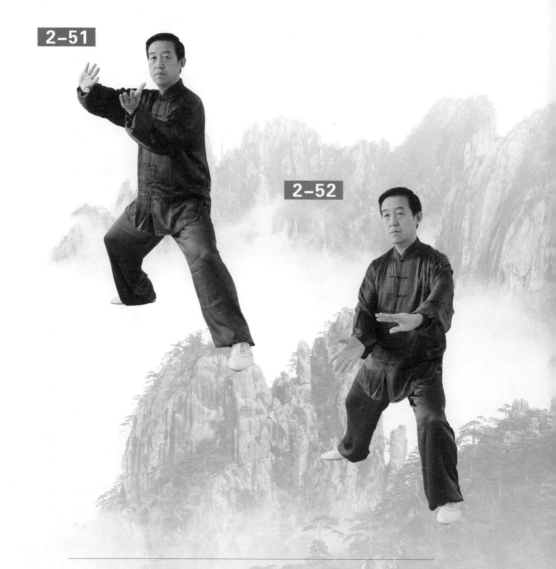

2-51

2-52

氣宜直養而無害
上下相隨妙無窮

Section Three
Steps Training Methods

1. Forward step exercises

1 Stand upright with your feet placed together. The body should be relaxed with your breathing and concentration focused into the Dantian. Eyes look forward. (Fig 2-53)

2 Shift the weight to the right leg and take a step forward-left with the left foot. At the same time, move both palms in a forward and upward arc. Then move both palms back in a counter clockwise motion with the left palm facing up and the right palm facing out. (Fig 2-54)

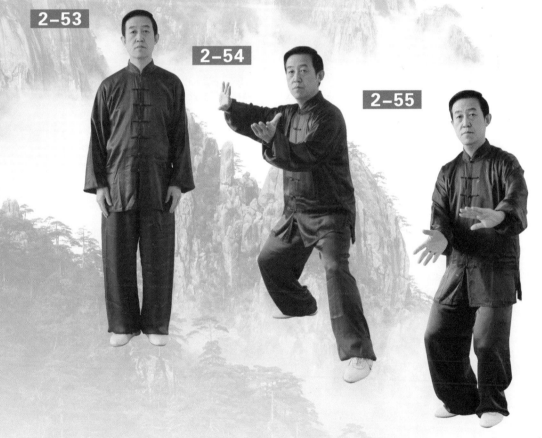

2-53

2-54

2-55

3 Continuing from the previous movement shift the weight to the left leg and draw the right foot to the inside of the left foot. At the same time, move both palms down and forward with both arms rotating clockwise so that the left palm is facing forward and the right palm is facing down. Eyes look forward. (Fig 2-55)

Take a step forward with the left foot and move both palms forward and upward in an arc then pull back to the same position as previous movement (Fig 2-54), so that the movements of the hands are well co-ordinated with the foot.

Repeat the exercise several times, and then repeat the exercise on the right side as mirrored movement. Take a step with the right foot and draw up the left foot. The essential points of the exercise are the same as the previous movement, with left and right reversed.

2. Backward step exercise

1 Stand upright with both feet close together. Eyes look forward. Rest the right palm on the right side of the waist. Raise left arm up high as your shoulder level and push the left palm forward, (centre of palm facing outwards) the elbow lowered and the shoulders relaxed. (Fig 2-56)

2 Continue from the previous movement. Shift your weight to the right leg, left foot steps in an arc to the rear-left, the ball of the left

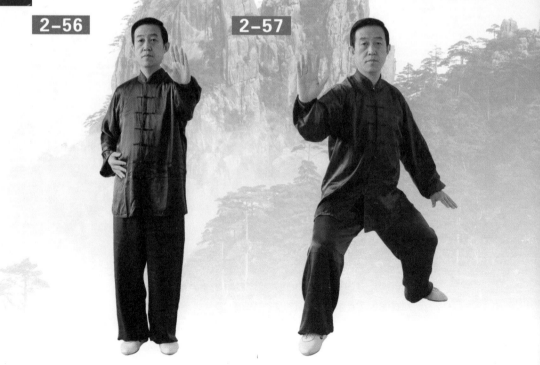

2-56   2-57

Foot sliding on the floor. At the same time, following the stepping back of the left foot, move the left palm down and back in an arc with the arm rotating clockwise slightly at the same time. Move the right palm back and turn it over whilst moving the palm up high as the shoulder so the palm faces forwards, then push it forward. (Fig 2-57)

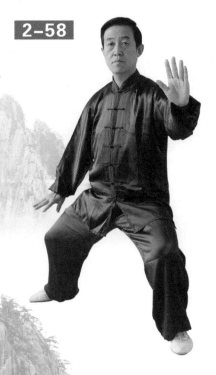

2-58

3 Continue from the previous movement. Shift the weight to the left leg, then the right foot steps in an arc to the rear right side past the inside of the left foot, the ball of the right foot sliding on the floor during the step movement. At the same time, following the stepping backward of the right foot, move the right palm down and back in an arc with right arm rotates counter clockwise. Move the left palm back and up turning it over whilst moving the palm up as high as shoulder so that it faces forwards. Then push it forward. (Fig 2-58)

The movements are a method to train the co-ordination of the upper and lower limbs in stepping back.

圍連滑轉　舒筋活血

3. Side step exercise

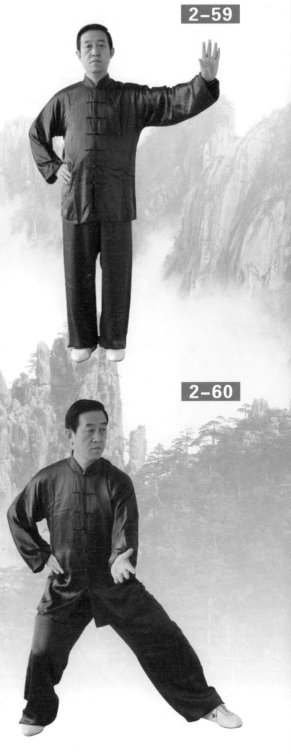

2-59

1 Stand upright with the feet placed together. Place the right palm on the right side of the waist with the thumb pointing back and the rest of the fingers forwards. Move the left palm to the left side of the body with the palm facing left forward high as shoulder with the shoulder relaxed and elbow lowered. Eyes look forward. (Fig 2-59)

2 Continue from the previous movement. Turn the body slightly to the right, shifting your weight to the right leg, lift the left foot up and take a step left with the left foot and place heel on the floor. At the same time move the left palm downward and rightward in an arc, with arm rotating counter clockwise. Eyes look forward-left. (Fig 2-60)

2-60

3 Continuing from the previous movement. Turn the body slightly to the left, shift the weight to the left foot, lift the right leg and draw the right foot to the inside of the left foot. At the same time, move the left palm to the right and upward to a shoulder level then push to leftward in an arc with the arm rotating clockwise so that the palm faces out at the end of the movement. Eyes look forward-left. (Fig 2-61)

This exercise is a method of training the co-ordination of the upper and lower body, by opening and closing the hand and foot in reverse order. Repeat this exercise for the Right side as well. Take a step rightward, the essential points of the exercise being the same as described above, simply reversing left and right. (Fig 2-62, 2-63, 2-64)

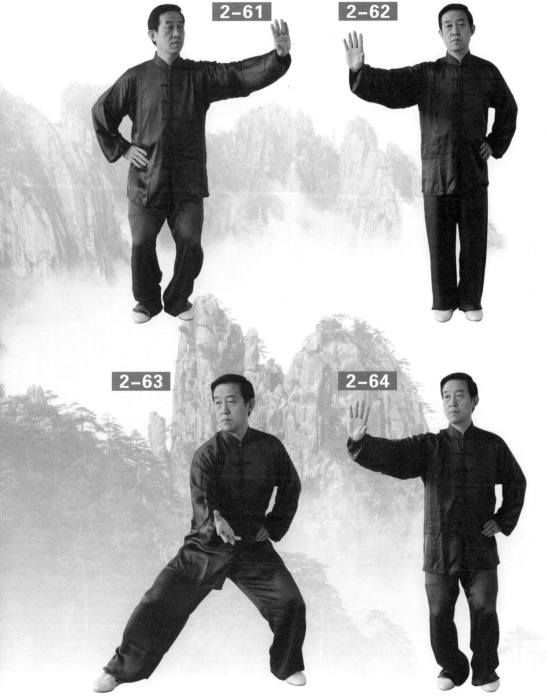

2-61

2-62

2-63

2-64

4. Wave hands incorporating footwork exercise

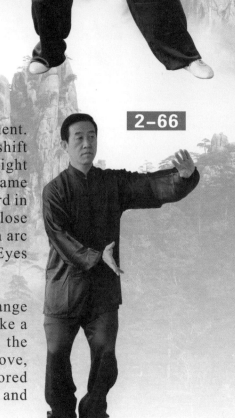

2-65

1 Stand upright with your feet together. Hang both arms naturally downward at the sides of the body, with the entire body relaxed. Eyes look forward. Relax the right hip, turn the body slightly to the right, keep the weight on the right leg, lift the left foot and take a step leftward with the heel of left foot landing on the floor, the toes of the foot lifted upwards. At the same time, move the right palm leftward and upward with the arm rotating counter clockwise and then ward it off upward and rightward. Move the left palm forward to the front of the abdomen so it is facing right. Eyes look forward-left. (Fig 2-65)

2-66

2 Continue from the previous movement. Turn the body slightly to the left and shift the weight on the left leg. Draw the right foot to the inside of the left foot. At the same time, move the left palm upward and leftward in an arc with the arm rotating clockwise. Close the right palm downward and leftward in an arc in front of the abdomen so it is facing left. Eyes look forward-left. (Fig 2-66)

Repeat this movement eight times then change this movement to the other side as well. Take a step rightward, the essential points of the exercise being the same as described above, simply reversing left and right as mirrored movement. The footwork should be light and natural.

5. Wave hands with feet in back cross-step exercise

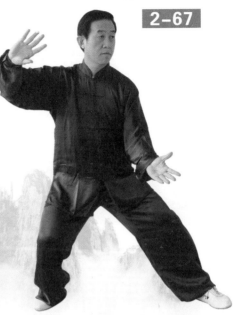

2-67

1 Stand upright with your feet together. Hang both arms naturally downward at the sides of the body, with the entire body relaxed. Eyes look forward. Relax the right hip, turn the body slightly to the right, shifting your weight to your right foot, lift the left leg and take a step leftwards with the heel of the left foot landing on the floor and the toes lifted upward. At the same time, move the right palm left and up as high as the shoulder with the arm rotating counter clockwise. Move the left palm forward to the front of the abdomen so that it is facing right. Eyes look forward-left. (Fig 2-67)

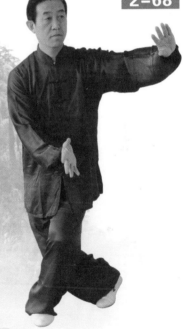

2-68

2 Continue from the previous movement. Move the right palm down and left in an arc until it is in front of the abdomen, rotate the arm clockwise so that the palm faces left. Move the left palm up and left until it is in front of the left shoulder. With the arm rotating clockwise so that the palm faces out to the left. At the same time, take a step to the rear-left of the left foot with the right foot. The ball of the right foot landing on the floor. Eyes look forward-right. (Fig 2-68)

3 Turn the body slightly to the right with the right palm moving left and up in an arc and rotate the arm counter clockwise so that the palm faces out to the right. Move the left palm down and left in an arc then cross to the front of the abdomen, with the arm rotating counter clockwise smoothly so that the palm faces right. At the same time, shift the weight on the right leg, lift the left foot up and take a step leftward with the heel of the foot landing on the floor and the toes lifted upward. Eyes look forward-left of the body. Return the movement to the position shown in Fig 2-67 and repeat this movement. You can do it for the right side as well. Take a step rightward, the essential points of the exercise being the same as described above, simply reversing left and right as mirrored movement.

Chapter Three
The Taiji Skills of Preserving Energy

The Taiji skill of preserving energy (Qigong) includes Sitting Quietly (meditation in a seated position), the Taiji Stance for energy collection and exercises lying down (these are not included in this book). Regardless of which method you use, they all relax the body, loosen the limbs, concentrate the spirit and centre your mind. It will enable you to discover your potential energy source and maintain your energy levels, keeping your metabolism rate and digestive system in a healthy state. It can also help you to control your temper and emotional states by reducing your levels of anxiety and stress. With Taiji Qigong, blood circulation improves and energy channels open. This gives better energy circulation which will help you to maintain a good healthy body, prolonging life and preserving mental faculties into later life.

Section One
Sitting–Quietly Method (Meditation)

1. Preparation before meditating

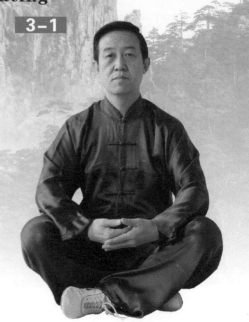

3-1

Preferably you should wear loose comfortable clothes. First practice the warm up exercises, as described in Chapter Two of the book, to let your muscles and tendons relax, helping your blood and Qi to circulate freely. While you are sitting, your back should be straight without leaning forward or back. Make sure the air in the area you practice is fresh and if you are indoors that it circulates freely leaving a window slightly ajar. However avoid strong currents of wind while you practice, and try to keep away from any external interruptions, such as phones or other people.

2. The posture of meditation

Sitting freely

Sit on the floor. If the floor is too hard sit on a stool or cushion. Cross your legs naturally, with your knees not flat on the floor. Try to be in a comfortable position facing south. Keep both arms in a circle and remain relaxed, with your palms on top of one another, facing upwards, and the right palm above the left one. (Fig. 3-1)

Sitting flatly

Sit on a chair or a wide bench with both feet placed on the floor as wide as your shoulders. Keep the knees at an angle of 90 degrees. Place both palms on top of your thighs, near to the knees, with palms facing up, (Fig. 3-2) or down. (Fig. 3-3) Close your eyes lightly or keep them open. While you are sitting, keep your head erect and your neck relaxed, your body upright in a balanced position. Do not lean forward, back, left or right. Tuck your chin in and close your mouth with your teeth touching lightly and the tip of your tongue lightly touching the upper palette. Relax your face muscles, keeping a serene expression. Shoulders, arms, elbows and wrists should be relaxed. Keep your chest relaxed and in a little. Your back, while you tuck your chest in a little, should stretch out slightly, maintaining an upright and relaxed position. Your lower abdomen (Dantian) should be loosened and settled, with the perineum (Huiyin) lifted up slightly (the Huiyin is located between the genitals and the anus).

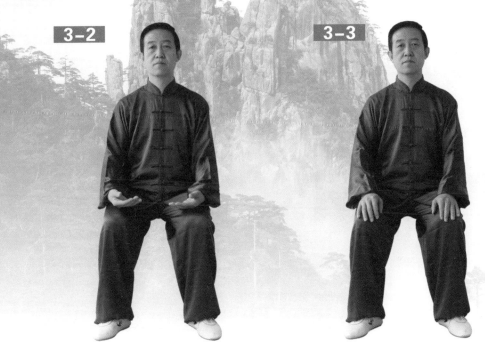

3-2 3-3

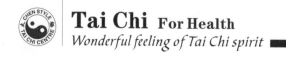
3. The key points of the exercise

Breathing naturally, whilst concentrating your mind

When your mind and body posture are relaxed and in position, focus on the movement of your breathing into your lower abdomen. Your breathing should be smooth, soft and natural. At the beginning, in order to speed up the energy collection, you could just simply use deep breaths, not worrying about focusing your mind on the exercise in great detail. Concentrate on your breathing, which should be controlled yet relaxed and as calm as possible, also try to focus your hearing to the back of your head. While you breath out, the focus of your mind should sink down from your heart to your lower abdomen, which will enable the heart energy to sink down to the Dantian. Constant practice in this way will gradually increase the heat in the Dantian. When you feel plenty of heat down in the Dantian, you should stop concentrating energy down to your lower abdomen in this way. Let the focus of your mind gently move away, whilst still breathing in and out from your Dantian (to maintain the heat and energy).

While you practice this Qigong, your mind should focus lightly on your Dantian. Do not be too frustrated nor persistent with your concentration. If you are more lightly and quietly focused on your Dantian, it will be easier for the energy to flow down to your lower abdomen and run throughout your body. If your mind is too tense and stressed, or if you are in a hurry for a quick result, the energy won`t flow freely through your body. As the ancient Chinese book of Qigong philosophy Neijing says, "with light focus and no intention, your internal energy will follow your mind." The more relaxed the body is and the calmer the mind is, the stronger the energy will be and the better it will circulate throughout your body.

Constant practice and gradual progression

When you first begin to practice this meditation use natural breaths combining the lungs with the lower abdomen at the same time. In accordance with the improvements of your Qigong, gradually begin to use only your lower abdomen, with long, soft, deep and smooth breaths. To develop this type of breathing takes time, and it is not easy or recommended for beginners to attempt this stage straight away. Beginners should not try to hold their breath to increase its length, longer breathing comes from longer practice. Naturally people breathe 12 to 40 times a minute, which is the recommended number for beginners to start with. With more experience this will gradually reduce to 2 or 3 times a minute. Beginners should be cautious with this type of exercise and should breathe according to their level of fitness.

Relieve stress and empty your mind

Randomly thinking of things or being anxious will disturb your Qigong practice. It will become easier for you to overcome these kinds of problems as your level of Qigong improves and you become more experienced. It is hard for beginners but this book will introduce some useful methods to help you relieve stress and empty your mind.

A) Counting breath

Count your breaths during your meditation. Start from number one onwards. With this method, concentrate on one thing, counting, so that every other thought in your mind disappears. After a while this one thing will disappear and you will be able to concentrate on your practice.

B) Convince yourself

While practicing meditation it is quite common to think about lots of things going on in your life. When this happens, you should tell yourself in your mind "I am practicing meditation now and any other things will wait for me to finish my practice. It is pointless to think about them now. I should relax, not worry and concentrate on my practice." Say this to yourself a few times until all other thoughts go away.

C) Clear your mind

When practicing meditation some people may find that they have too many thoughts and worries in their mind. This may result in some peoples` minds creating images of what they are thinking or worrying about. If this happens and you feel uncomfortable or scared, you should open your eyes and let the image disappear. This kind of image is caused by your own mind, because you are thinking of something too much. For example, if you are looking forward to visiting somewhere and are constanly thinking about it, you may see that place while you are meditating. In that case the best way to get rid of an image of that kind is to clear your mind, have a short break and then continue practicing.

Put emphasis on the Dantian naturally

After a period of practicing meditation the inside and the surface of your body may experience various sensations such as cold, hot, light, heavy, solid, tingling, bulging or tickling. Initially, the tip of your fingers and your feet will be the likeliest place to get these kinds of feeling. Then the stomach and the intestines may possibly experience some sensations, with your body or part of your body feeling cool on the surface and warmer inside. Some muscles may begin to shake and feel tingly. All these feelings depend on the individual with some people experiencing strong sensations and others simply feeling relaxed and calm. Sometimes images may appear in a similar way to when your mind is thinking too much. These can range from a mountain or a lake to even a person. In this case you should not be concerned. Also you should not be very anxious to see these kinds of images, because they are not real, they are a creation of your mind.

As those kinds of images occur, you should keep your mind still not paying attention to them. Focus on your Dantian. Let the image disappear itself. In Chinese we say: "Treat strange things as not strange. Then the strange things will become normal." All these kinds of images will disappear and your mind will gradually become cleared as your level of meditation improves. The perfect stage of meditation is when no thoughts remain in your mind and it is as still as water with long, deep, smooth and continuous breaths, naturally coming only from the lower abdomen. Your mind will drift between being completely absorbed in the moment or absolute concentration.

4. Completing exercise

With both palms touch your Dantian and start to rotate them as if you were brushing the area. Move them in a circle 36 times in a clockwise direction. Start from the centre of your Dantian and then enlarge the cirles to your chest area. Reverse the motion back to your Dantian for 24 circles. After that, rub both palms together quickly and then massage your face with your palms 12 times. This kind of exercise is good for the spleen. After that, cross the back of your thumbs and rub them together. Use the back of the thumbs to massage your eyebrows and the area below the eyes 12 times. This exercise helps to maintain healthy eyesight. After that place both palms on top of and behind your ears using them to fold your ears over. The middle fingers of your palms should be connected behind your head at the mid-section of your skull. Lock your index fingers on top of your middle fingers, and use them to bang the cavity at the back of your head (Fengfu) for 36 times. This exercise is good for your hearing and the energy circulation from your body to your head. After that use both palms to massage from your thighs down to your ankles. Stand up slowly to finish your exercise.

Attention:

Although you should practice hard and treat this exercise seriously and carefully, do not be anxious for a quick result. As ancient Chinese philosophy says: "You should not be anxious to feel something in your mind and there should be no temptation to feel something. If you place your mind too heavily onto something, you will perceive the illusion of that something. If you have no temptation, you will not get anything. If you want to achieve something, drift between concentration and no concentration, and it will always be there." In conclusion, relax, enjoy, do not worry, avoid becoming anxious and try to practice regularly without pushing yourself too hard. Have the motivation to practice but try not to focus on the end result.

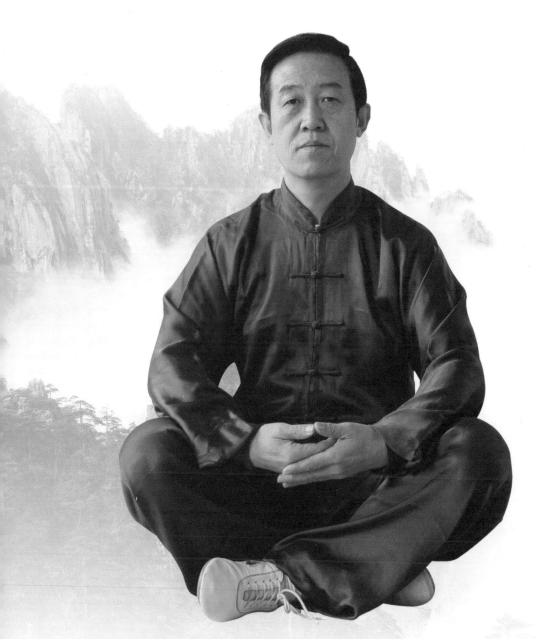

太極 養生功

Grandmaster Chen Zhenglei in Meditation pictures.

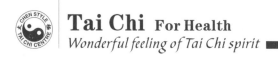

Section Two
Energy Collection Exercise

1. The method of increasing energy

1 Place both feet shoulder-width apart, toes turned outwards slightly. Bend your knees and keep your hips relaxed, sitting down a little from your hips. Keep your body upright and your head erect naturally. Keep your chest and chin in and lower your waist. Relax all parts of your body, with your arms by your side, in a natural stance. Your palms should be open with your fingers straight and relaxed without tension, facing your thighs. Close both eyes lightly and look inside as if you can see your Dantian. Your teeth and lips should be touching each other gently, and your tongue should be gently touching your upper palette. Breathe naturally. (Fig 3-4)

2 Carry on from the previous position. Rotate both palms outwards and raise both arms up to ear level, with elbows bending slightly. Breath in during this movement. (Fig 3-5)

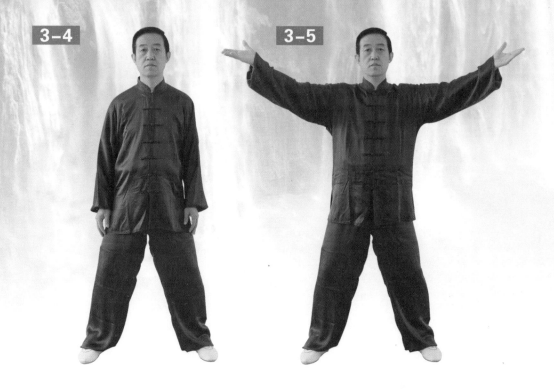

3-4

3-5

3 Raise your arms above your head, with the elbows bent and your palms facing the top of your head (the arm movement should be in a circular motion from the starting position). Keep breathing in until the end of the movement. (Fig 3-6)

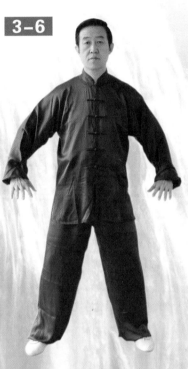

3-6

4 Sink your body down slightly. Following the sinking of your body, your palms should press down to the Dantian. (Fig 3-7) As you press down, your arms and shoulders should be relaxed. Keep your palms in front of your Dantian for a few seconds and then separate them to your side, as in the starting position. Breathe out during this movement, and imagine the Qi sinking down to the bottom of your feet (Yongquan). (Fig 3-8)

5 As you return your arms to the starting position, repeat the whole movement from the beginning, as many times as you like (preferably more than 8). This exercise will enable you to initiate your energy circulation and achieve a stronger Qi feeling.

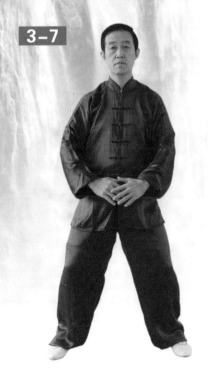

3-7

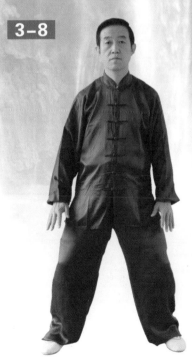

3-8

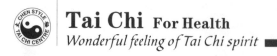
Key to the movement:
While you practice you should keep your breathing deep, long, smooth and gentle. It may not be easy for beginners to do so, but try to concentrate on your breathing as much as possible following the movement in and out. While you breathe in, imagine that both your arms, as they open, are collecting the energy from space and earth to your Baihui (central point on the top of your head). As you breath out, imagine the energy flowing down from your Baihui to your Dantian. Keep it there for a few seconds (while your palms are in front of your Dantian). From your Dantian the energy flows down to Huiyin (perineum) and from there it splits and is delivered through both the inside of your legs, down to Yong Quan (central point at the sole of your feet). By this way you can maintain a very good energy level and get rid of the negative energy in your body and fortify yourself against disease and sickness.

2. The method of grasping the energy

1 Stand upright with feet together and toes turned outward slightly. Bend your knees and keep your hips relaxed, sitting down a little from your hips. Keep your body upright and your head erect naturally. Keep your chest and chin in and lower your waist. Relax all parts of your body, with your arms by your side, in a natural stance. Breathe naturally and look forward. (Fig 3-9)

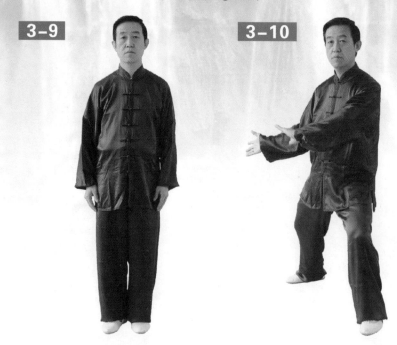

3-9
3-10

2 Raise the left foot, breathing in. Step diagonally forward with your left foot, breathing out as you go, to form a Bow stance shifting your weight onto the front (left) leg, whilst bending your right knee. Lift both arms forward and up in a circle. Eyes look forward. (Fig 3-10)

3 Change both palms into fists and at the same time shift your weight backwards in a circle. Imagine as if you are grabbing the energy pulling it down and backwards. Look forward and breathe in. (Fig 3-11, 3-12)

4 Change both fists into palms and push forward in an upward circle. Breathe out. (Fig 3-13) Repeat this exercise from step 3 (Fig 3-11) 8 times.

Key to the movement:
You can repeat this movement on the right side as well, with the right foot stepping forward diagonally instead of the left. The rest of the movement is the same as above. The most important aspect of this movement is to shift your weight between your legs smoothly in a natural circular motion. Also let your Dantian connect with your Mingmen (the center of your lower back) so that they work together, as a unit.

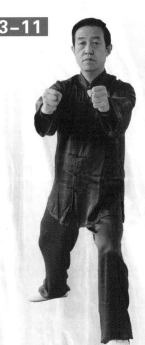

3-11

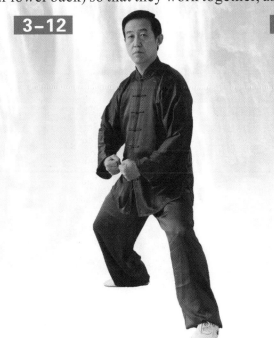

3-12

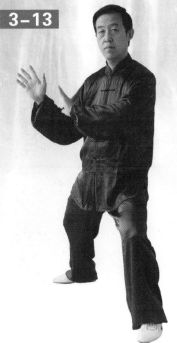

3-13

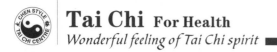
3. Rotate the energy in the Dantian

1 Place both feet shoulder width apart, with toes turned outward slightly. Bend your knees and keep your hips relaxed, sitting down from your hips a little. Keep your body upright and your head naturally erect. Keep your chest and chin in and lower your waist. Relax every part of your body, with your left palm gently touching your navel, and your right palm covering the left one. Gently close both eyes and look inside as if you can see your Dantian. Your teeth and lips should be gently touching each other, and your tongue should be gently touching your upper palette. Breathe naturally. (Fig 3-14)

2 Men start rotating your palms clockwise, women anticlockwise around navel in a circle. Begin with small circles and gradually enlarge them, expanding the circles around your chest and your lower abdomen. Complete a total of 36 circles. then, change the position of both palms, with the left covering the right, and start rotating them counter clockwise in the same circling motion for 24 times. Start with big circles around your chest and lower abdomen, and finish with small ones around your navel. (Fig 3-15, 3-16)

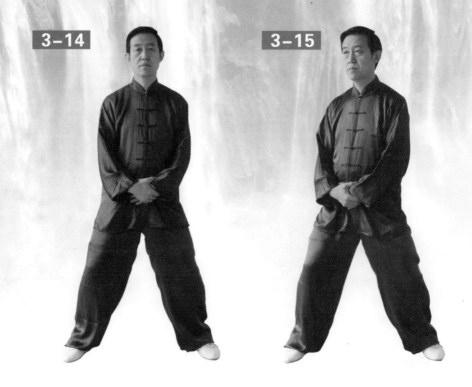

3-14

3-15

While you rotate your hands, your weight should follow the movement of the hands accordingly. You should also include your body in the movement by turning it to both sides in opposition to the weight movement (for example, if you shift your weight on your right leg, your body should turn to left slightly).

Attention: For women the position of the palms and the rotating direction should be opposite to what is described above. Begin with the right palm on top of your navel, and the left palm covering the right. Start rotating counter clockwise for 36 times. Then change the position of the palms (the left one covering the right one) and rotate clockwise for 24 times.

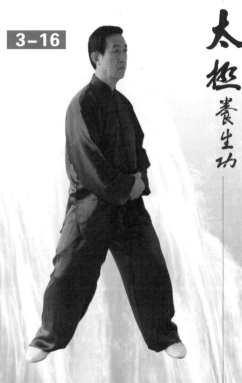

3-16

4. Taiji Hunyuan Stance

1 Place both feet shoulder-width apart, with toes turned outwards slightly. Bend knees and keep hips relaxed, sitting down a little from hips. Keep body upright and head naturally erect. Keep chest

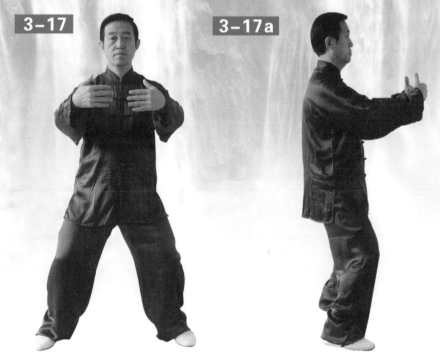

3-17   3-17a

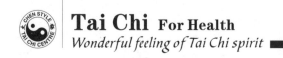
and chin in and lower waist. Relax every part of your body, with arms held in a circle in front of chest and palms facing your body. Keep fingers relaxed and naturally straight. Bend elbows and drop them down slightly. Keep the head erect and the body naturally upright. Lightly focus the mind on a feeling of rising up through the top of the head (the crown, Baihui). Close both eyes slightly and look inside as if you can see your Dantian. Your teeth and lips should be gently touching each other, and your tongue should be gently touching your upper palette.

Both thighs should form a kind of 'rounded bridge' position. Both feet should be placed firmly on the floor with the outer edge of the sole and the heel feeling as if they were grabbing it. Keep the centre of the feet (Yongquan) lifted lightly and place your body weight exactly onto the centre of your feet. (Fig 3-17, 3-17a)

Key to the movement:
Concentrate your mind and focus on the exercise. Relax your whole body and let your internal energy flow inside your body naturally. The breathing requirements should be the same as in Chapter 3, Section One, part 3: The key points of exercising.

5. Completing exercise

Same as Chapter 3, Section One, part 4: Completing exercise on page 62

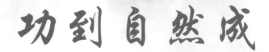

Chapter Four
Illustration of The 18 Forms
of Chen Style Tai Chi

Section One
Names of the Movements

Form 1 Preparing Form

Form 2 Buddha's Warrior Attendant Pounds Mortar

Form 3 Lazy About Tying the Coat

Form 4 Six Sealing and Four Closing

Form 5 Single Whip

Form 6 White Crane Spreads Its Wings

Form 7 Walk Diagonally

Form 8 Brush Knee

Form 9 Stepping to Both Sides (Three Steps Forward)

Form 10 Cover hands and Strike with Fist

Form 11 High Pat on the Horse

Form 12 Kick with the Left Heel

Form 13 Jade Girl Works at Shuttles

Form 14 Wave Hands

Form 15 Turn Body with Double Lotus Kick

Form 16 Cannon Fist Over Head

Form 17 Buddha's Warrior Attendant Pounds Mortar

Form 18 Finishing Form

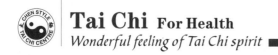

Section Two
Illustrated Instruction of the Movements

Form 1 – Preparing Form

1 Stand naturally upright with the feet together. Let both arms hang by the sides of the body, with the palms facing inward beside the thighs. Keep the head erect. Close the mouth lightly with the tongue gently touching the upper palate. Look straight ahead. (Figure 4-1)

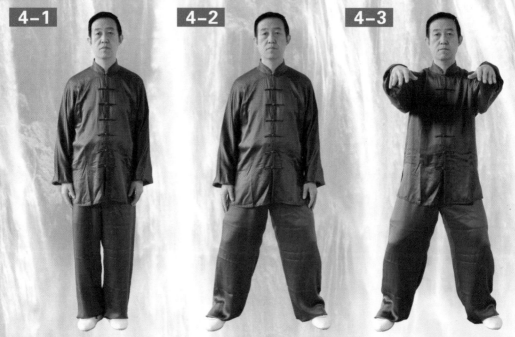

2 Bend both knees and relax the hips whilst sinking the body. Lift the left foot up and step out to the left, just a little wider than shoulder-width. Place the toe down first and then the whole foot. In this position both feet should be turned slightly outward and in firm contact with the ground. The arch of the foot (Yong Quan point) should be lifted lightly and free from the floor with the weight centered evenly through the feet. The body is relaxed, the chest slightly sunk, the shoulders relaxed, the weight rooted and the elbows dropped. Keep the head erect and the body naturally upright. Lightly focus the mind on a feeling of rising up through the top of the head (the crown). The eyes look straight ahead. (Figure 4-2)

Key requirements to the movement:

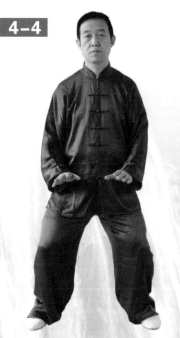

4-4

When stepping out to the left, the weight must first be transferred onto the right leg, then the left foot can be lifted in a controlled manner. As you move out to the left the toes contact the ground first, and then gradually through the foot to the heel. Transfer your weight across slowly.

The entire body relaxes and the internal energy (Qi) flows down to the Dantian (lower abdomen) then through the legs down to the Yong Quan point on the sole of the foot. While bending the knees and relaxing the hips, breathe out deeply as the body is sinking down. Mentally relax and calm down whilst retaining a concentrated spirit and consciousness. Think of nothing and try to achieve a state of Wuji, which is the state where there is no yin and yang division. This is the state that exists before Taiji. Taiji comes from Wuji.

3 Raise both arms up slowly to shoulder level, with both palms facing down. Keep the shoulders relaxed and the elbows slightly bent. The knees and hips are relaxed and as the arms rise up, the body sinks down slightly. Both feet remain firmly on the floor. The eyes look straight ahead. (Figure 4-3)

Key requirements to the movement:
As the arms rise up and the body sinks down, the muscles of the chest, back, waist, ribs and abdomen must be relaxed. Do not let the shoulders rise up with the arms. Breathe in through the nose and do not hold the breath.

4 As the body relaxes, it sinks down slowly from the hips and the knees bend slightly as well. The shoulders and the elbows relax, the arms draw in slightly towards the body with the elbows bent slightly and both hands press downward until they are in front of the lower abdomen with the palms facing downwards. (Figure 4-4)

Key requirements to the movement:
Whilst pressing down do not use tension, keep the movement relaxed. The body sinks down through use of the hips, knees and ankles so that the body remains upright. Do not lean from the waist! This position should look as if you are sitting on a chair. Exhale as you lower your hands and the body sinks. (Breathe out through the nose)

Form 2 Buddha's Warrior Attendant Pounds Mortar

1 Turn the upper body to the left slightly and shift the weight on to the right leg. Turn both palms in a clockwise direction and raise the arms so that the left hand has the palm facing outward and is located above the left knee at eye level. The right hand palm, facing up, is in front of the chest on the centre line of the body. Eyes look forward and left. (Figure 4-5)

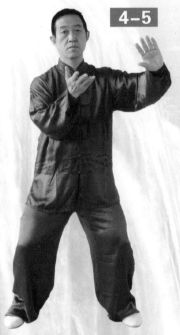
4-5

Key requirements to the movement:
Whilst turning the body and moving both palms up, relax and sink the hips. Co-ordinate the hips and the waist to utilize their combined strength and let this strength extend to both palms. Breathe in during this movement.

2 Move the body weight onto the left leg and relax the left hip, turn the hands in an anti-clockwise direction so that the left palm changes to face diagonally upwards and the right palm changes to face outwards. Turn the body 90 degrees to the right, lifting the toes of the right foot. At the same time the hands follow the body movement towards the right. Eyes look forward. Breathe out during this movement. (Figure 4-6)

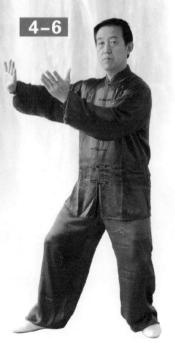
4-6

3 Sink and shift the weight onto the right leg and lift the left foot up with the knee bent. Bend the right knee and relax the hip, the upper body sinks down and turns to the right, both palms keep pushing upward and outward; eyes look left forward. (Figure 4-7)

Key requirements to the movement:
Sinking the upper body must be co-ordinated with lifting the left foot. Don`t bend the waist and protrude the buttocks. Breathe in during this movement.

4 Move the left foot out forward-left with the heel sliding along the floor, the toes lifted up and turned inward; Keep the weight on the right leg with both palms pushing to the rear-right, in an upward and outward direction. Transfer the weight from the right leg onto the left leg. The whole left foot is placed on the floor with the toes turned outward slightly. (Figure 4-8) Eyes look to the left and forward.

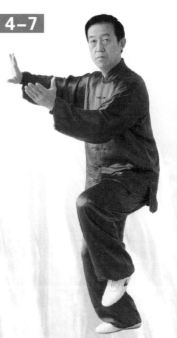

4-7

Key requirements to the movement:
Keep the torso upright whilst the left foot slides diagonally forward, both palms push diagonally toward the back right. This forms a cross co-ordinated line of strength. Breathe out during this movement.

5 Whilst transferring the weight, turn the upper body to the left about 45 degrees, both palms move down and forward in an arc with both arms rotating clockwise. The left palm moves to the front of the left side of the chest, with the elbow bent and the palm facing downward. The right palm moves down in front of the right leg above the knee, with the palm facing outward and fingers pointing behind. Eyes look forward. (Figure 4-9)

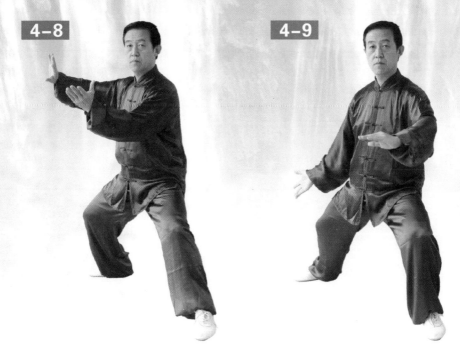

4-8

4-9

Key requirements to the movement:

Turning of the body, shifting the weight and moving the palms should be co-ordinated. Keep the pelvis down and move the hips forward. The left arm maintains a circular structure and keeps the 'Peng' (outward push) strength throughout. Keep the right elbow about 8 to 10 centimeters away from the body. The left knee should align vertically above the left ankle. Do not let the knee protrude forward. The right knee is bent and the hips are relaxed. Maintain an arched structure to the legs throughout the movement. Breathe in at the beginning and out at the end of this movement.

6 Keeping the body weight on the left leg, step (move) the right leg forward placing the toes on the ground to create an `empty stance` (no weight on the right leg). At the same time the right hand follows the right leg in a forward rising arc with the palm facing upward in front of the right side of the chest. The fingers of the left hand lightly touch the right forearm. Eyes look forward. (Figure 4-10)

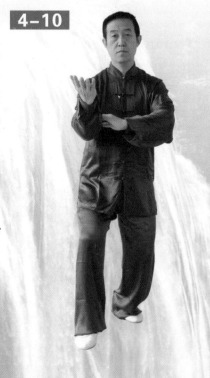

4-10

Key requirements to the movement:

The right foot steps forward with the knees bent and the hips relaxed with light, flexible and natural footwork. The movement of the arms co-ordinates with the rise and fall of the body. Breathe in during this movement.

7 The left palm turns upwards and sinks down to the front of the lower abdomen. At the same time the right hand forms a fist. Lower the back of the fist into the opened left palm. Eyes look forward. (Figure 4-11)

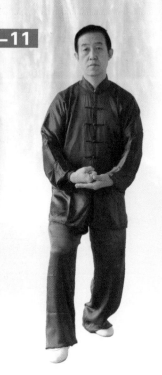

4-11

Key requirements to the movement:
Keep both hands and the abdomen about 8 to 10 cm. apart, both arms hold a feeling of rounded outward 'Peng' strength. The waist sinks down as the fist lowers into the left palm. Breathe out during this movement.

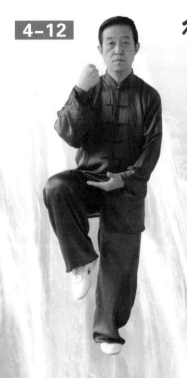

4-12

8 Raise the right fist up to shoulder level in front of the body and at the same time, lift the right knee whilst maintaining relaxed hips and a bent left knee. The right toes point naturally downward and the lower leg is turned slightly inward to a position close to the left knee. Eyes look forward. (Figure 4-12)

Key requirements to the movement:
As the right hand and foot rise up, the left side sinks down. (One side of the body is in yin, the other is in yang.) Do not rise up on the supporting leg as the right knee lifts. The internal energy flows down along the body. As the fist rises, the shoulders stay relaxed and the right elbow is dropped down. Breathe in during this movement.

4-13

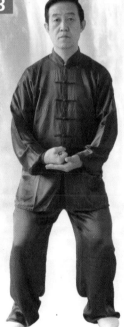

9 Stamp the right foot on the floor about shoulder-width apart from left foot and place it firmly on the floor. At the same time the back of the right fist strikes downward onto the center of the left palm, both arms are bent and maintain a feeling of rounded outward 'Peng' strength. Eyes look forward. (Figure 4-13)

Key requirements to the movement:
Stamping the foot and pounding the right fist is a co-ordinated power releasing movement. Keep the knees bent and hips relaxed. The internal energy flows down to the Dantian. Breathe out during this movement.

Form 3 Lazy About Tying Coat

1 Turn the body slightly to the left and transfer the weight to the right leg. Change the right fist into a palm that moves to the left a little, then upward and right in a circle to the front right side of the head. Throughout this movement the right arm rotates counter clockwise and the left palm rotates clockwise to press down to the side of the left hip. Eyes look forward left. (Figure 4-14)

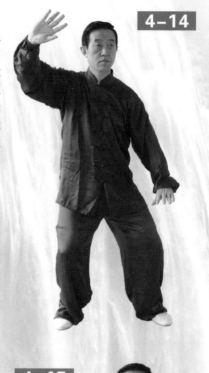
4-14

Key requirements to the movement:
In order to use the body to lead the arm movement, the waist should be sunk and should turn before the right palm pushes up in a circle. The right palm movement should be co-ordinated with the movement of the left palm pressing down to generate an `opening strength`. Breathe in slowly.

2 The right arm rotates clockwise and the palm moves a little to the right, then presses down in a circle across the front of the body. Finally bring the right arm in front of the left chest with the palm facing upward. The left palm pushes to the left then rotates up counter clockwise in a circle and crosses with the right arm in front of the chest. The left arm stays on top of the inner right forearm with left palm facing outward. Transfer the weight on to the left leg and lift the right foot up to take a large step out to the right. When the foot moves, keep the inside of the right heel sliding on the floor with the toes lifted and turned inward. Eyes look right. (Figure 4-15)

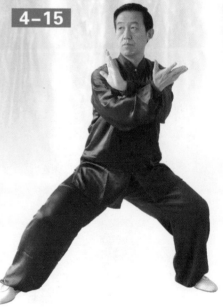
4-15

Key requirements to the movement:
The step out should be co-ordinated with the crossing of both arms in front of the chest and the arm and foot movements should occur simultaneously and finish at the same time. The step out should be very light, natural and sensitive. Breathe out during this movement.

3 Turn the upper body to the left and transfer the weight to the right. The right palm rotates clockwise then moves to the left a little and pushes upward. Eyes look right forward. (Figure 4-16)

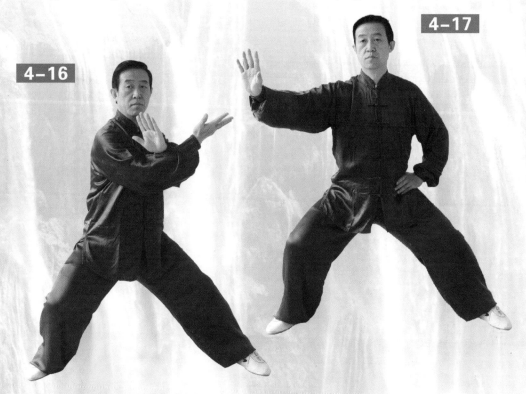

Key requirements to the movement:
When transferring the weight, the hips move in an arc to the rear. Maintain the 'outward push strength' through the left elbow and right arm keeping space between the arms and the body - the armpits should be free and in a rounded shape. Breathe in during this movement.

4 Turn the upper body to the right and rotate the right arm counter clockwise. The right palm pushes up and forward to the right in an arc to cross the front of the body until it is above the right knee with the fingers at eye level. The left palm rotates back slightly at the end of the movement and the body sinks down and turns back to the front. Keep the shoulders relaxed and the elbows lowered. The left arm rotates counter clockwise and moves down in a circle across the abdomen until it reaches the left side of the waist; then rotating clockwise put the left palm on the left side of your waist, with the thumb at the back and fingers at the front. The weight is on the right leg. Eyes follow the right hand during the movement then look forward at the end of movement. (Figure 4-17)

Key requirements to the movement:
When pushing the right palm, use the waist to lead the shoulder and shoulder to lead the elbow. Relax the shoulder, drop down the elbow and the wrist, to allow the strength to go through to the tips of fingers. The internal energy should be flowing throughout the waist, shoulders, arms and ultimately to the fingertips. In the final position, the hips and waist are relaxed, the groin open, the shoulders sunk down and the elbows low. More percentage of the weight is on the right side and less weight on the left side with the right knee over the right heel (do not over bend the knee). The left leg extends with the knee bent slightly and left toes turned inward. The torso is naturally upright free and comfortable. Breathe out during this movement.

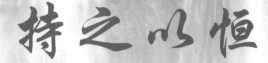

持之以恒

Form 4   Six Sealing and Four Closing

1 Turn your body to the right and transfer the weight slightly to that side. Move your left hand up in a circle until it is close to the right hand whilst at the same time the right arm follows the body to the right slightly and starts to press down a little. Eyes look at the tip of right middle figures. (Figure 4-18)

Key requirement to the movement:
When the left hand moves toward the right hand it should co-ordinate with the turning of the body and the weight transferring to the right. Both wrists sink and the fingers point up. Breathe in during this movement.

2 Turn the upper body to the left and transfer the weight on the left leg. Rollback both of the arms in an arc down and left rotating them clockwise until they reach waist level. Eyes look forward right. (Figure 4-19)

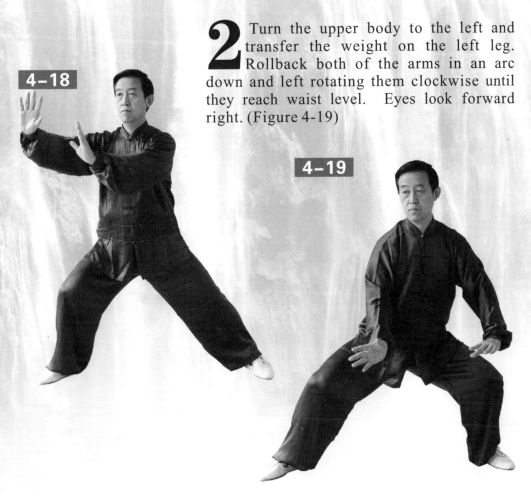

4-18

4-19

Key requirements to the movement:
As both arms rollback, sink the weight and use 'lu' and 'peng' energy (rollback and ward off). Breathe out during this movement.

3 Continue turning the body to the left rotating both arms clockwise. Both arms continue their arc left and up. Start to transfer the weight to the right slightly whilst the eyes look forward and left. (Figure 4-20)

Key requirements to the movement:
As both arms rollback, keep some weight in the right leg maintaining warding off strength throughout. Breathe in during this movement.

4 Without stopping from the previous movement, continue to transfer the weight to the right leg, and bring both palms up to the front of the left shoulder. Both palms face diagonally down and out. Turn the body to right slightly with the eyes look forward and right. (Figure 4-21)

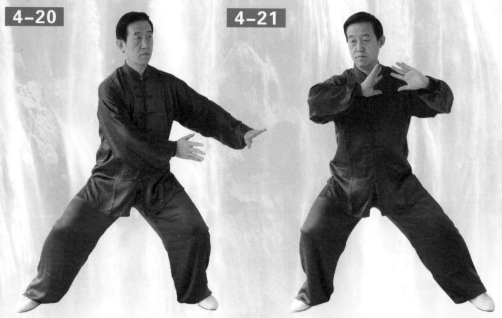

4-20   4-21

Key requirements to the movement:
When changing the hands from 'rollback strength' to 'palm pressing down strength', the movements of rollback are at the lower level while press down occurs at the higher level. These are led by a shift of the hips to the left followed by a turn of the waist to the right. The shoulders relax and the elbows sink down. Rotate the arms and wrists to turn the palms. Maintain 'warding off' strength without becoming stiff or too loose. Move and turn the body naturally, freely and smoothly. The in breath continues during this movement.

5 Keep the weight right and turn the body to the right whilst sinking down slightly. Combine the strength of both arms and press down both palms to the front right over the knee in a rounded action. Move the left foot into the inside of the right foot with a distance of approx. 20 centimeters with the left ball of the foot on the floor. Eyes look forward, slightly down and right . (figure 4-22)

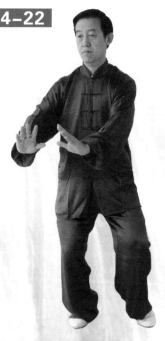

4-22

Key requirements to the movement:
As both palms press down, relax the hips and sink the weight. Relax the shoulders and drop the elbows to utilize their combined strength. The push co-ordinates with the body sinking. Breathe out during this movement.

Form 5 Single Whip

1 Turn the body to the right slightly and rotate the left arm toward the centerline of the body with the palm facing up and the fingers extending slightly forward. Rotate the right arm clockwise and pull the right palm backward slightly with the palm facing upward. Keeping the weight on the right leg. The left knee turns inward slightly using the toes on the floor as a pivot. Eyes look at both palms. (Figure 4-23)

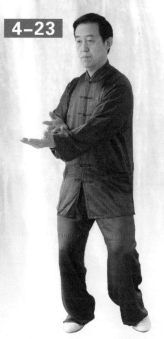

4-23

Key requirements to the movement:
Rotate both arms smoothly and freely, as opposed to just pulling back and pushing forward without rotation. Breathe in during this movement.

2 Turn the body to the left and keep the weight on the right leg. Turn the left leg out using the toes on the floor as a pivot. Close the fingertips of the right hand into a hook hand and extend it to the upper right until it is at shoulder level, with the fingertips pointing down. Draw the left hand to the front of the lower abdomen with the palm facing upwards. Maintain warding off strength on the left elbow. Eyes look at the right hand. (Figure 4-24)

4-24

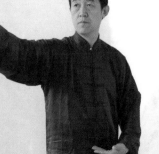

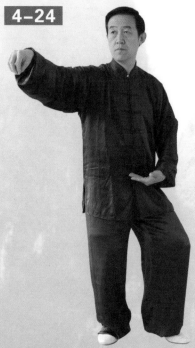

Key requirements to the movement:
As the body turns to the left, change the right palm to a hook, keep the weight sinking down, the shoulders relaxed and the elbows dropped down. Use the waist as an axis to initiate movements in the arms and hands. This movement is an opening posture with an out breath.

3 Turn the body to the right and transfer all the weight to the right leg, lift the left foot up with the left knee bent and turned in. Maintain the strength in the right wrist and keep the left palm steady, shoulders relaxed and elbows sunk down. Eyes look forward left. (Figure 4-25)

Key requirements to the movement:
The upper body should co-ordinate with the lower body. Keep the body upright and do not lean from the waist or protrude the buttocks. This movement is a closing posture with an in breath.

4 Stand on the right leg and move the left foot out to the left side with the inside of the sole sliding on the floor lightly. As the left foot slides out, the left toe points up and in. The right wrist maintains the upward strength and the left hand sinks down to form a counterbalance. Eyes look forward to the left. (Figure 4-26)

Key requirements to the movement:
Keep the body upright and never loose the warding off strength. This movement is an opening posture with an out breath.

4-25

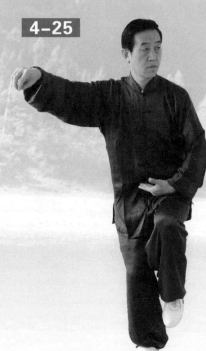

5 Turn the body to the right slightly and transfer the weight to the left leg to form a left bow step, thrust the left palm up to the right chest and rotate the arm inward. Eyes look forward to glance at the left palm. (Figure 4-27)

Key requirements to the movement:
When transferring the weight to the left, sink and move the hips in a rear arc whilst turning the body at the same time. The left knee should not be bent beyond the left toe. The shoulder and elbow should not be raised up when rotating the left arm. Breathe in during this movement.

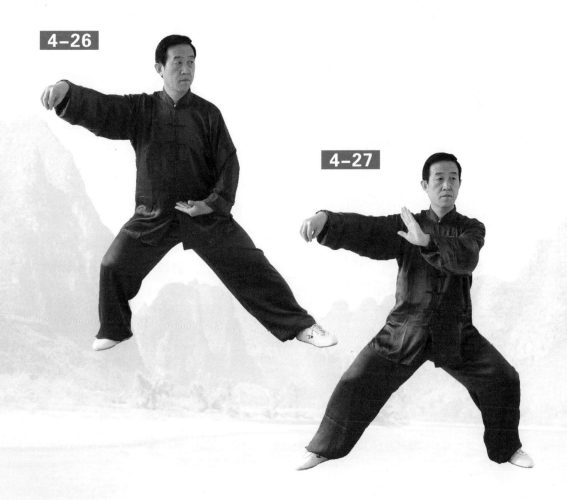

4-26

4-27

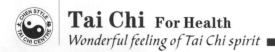

6 As the body turns left, slightly rotate the left arm clockwise and push the left palm forward and then to the left side of the body in a forward circle. As the left palm reaches the left side of the body sink the elbow with the arm aligned over the leg. The body weight sinks down at the same time. Eyes follow the left palm to the side of body then return to look forward. (Figure 4-28)

Key requirements to the movement:
Keep left toes outward and right toes inward, relax the hips and bend the knees. The body remains upright and the top of the head is held up at attention lightly. Relax the shoulders and sink the elbows. Upper and lower limbs co-ordinate to give the posture its strength. This movement combines an external body opening posture with an internal body closing posture with an out breath.

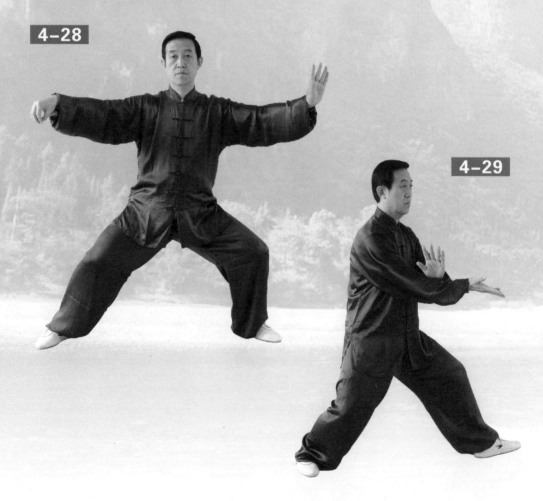

4-28

4-29

Form 6 White Crane Spreads Its Wings

1 Transfer the weight to the right leg and turn body to the left and turn the left toes out, change the right hook-hand into a palm and rotate the arm clockwise. Bring the left arm to the centre until both arms cross in front of the chest. Keep the left palm facing to the right with the fingers up and the right palm facing up with the fingers pointing forward. Eyes look forward and right. (Figure 4-29)

2 Turn the body to the left further and transfer the weight on to the left leg. Step the right foot forward diagonally. Rotate the right arm to chest centre and apply warding off strength. (Figure 4-30)

3 Turn the body to the right and transfer the weight to the right leg. From having both arms crossed and centered in front of the chest press the left palm down to hip level just above the left knee with the palm facing down. Simultaneously push the right palm up to the forward-right of the head with the palm facing out. Both of the arms form a circular structure. Draw the left foot to the forward-left of the right foot with the toes touching the floor. Eyes look forward. (Figure 4-31)

Key requirements to the movement:
Keep the stepping light and the left foot in an 'empty stance' with no weight on it. Keep the head erect, shoulders relaxed and body upright. Breathe in at the start and breathe out at the end.

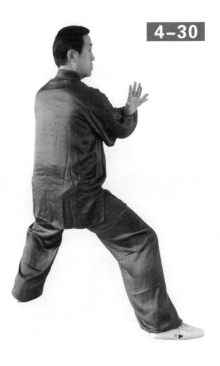

4-30

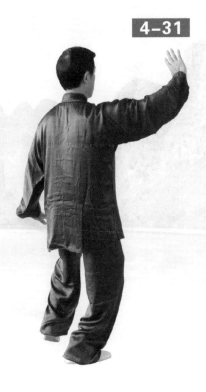

4-31

太極養生功

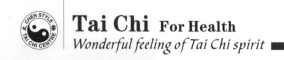
Form 7 Walk Diagonally

1 Keep the feet stationery and turn the body to the left. The left palm moves back and rotates clockwise whilst the right palm circles left and rotates clockwise. Keep the shoulders relaxed and the elbows down. Eyes look forward left. (Figure 4-32)

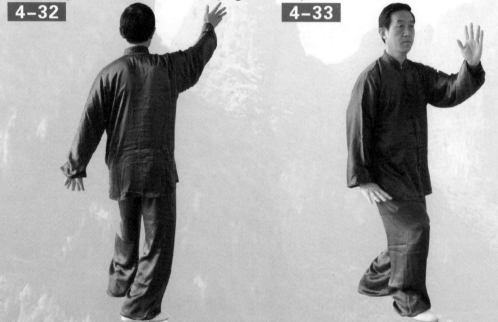

4-32

4-33

Key requirements to the movement:
The waving and rotating of the arms should be led by the body with a quality similar to wind lightly swaying the branches of a tree. Breathe in during this movement.

2 Put the left heel down on the floor and transfer the weight to the left foot whilst turning both the body and the right toes to the right. The left knee is bent and turned in slightly. As the body turns right the left hand circles to the centerline of the body in line with the nose with the palm facing right and the fingers up. At the same time rotate the right palm counter clockwise and press down to the right side of the thigh in a circle with palm facing down. Eyes look forward left. (Figure 4-33)

Key requirements to the movement:
Use the waist as a central axis and keep the head erect and the crown lifted. Breathe out during this movement.

3 Transfer the weight to the right leg and raise the left foot with a bent knee. Push both palms to the upward-right with warding off strength. Eyes look forward left. (Figure 4-34)

Key requirements to the movement:
As both palms push up, sink the body down slightly and root all the weight in the right leg, with relaxed hips and bent knees. The upper body should be co-ordinated with the lower body. Breathe in during this movement.

4 The body sinks further and the left foot takes a large step diagonally forward, sliding the inside heel along the floor with the toes up. Hold both arms up with 'warding off strength' throughout. Eyes look forward left. (Figure 4-35)

Key requirements to the movement:
As the left foot steps (diagonally forward), push both arms up with warding-off strength and sink the waist. The upper body should co-ordinate with the lower body. Breathe out during this movement.

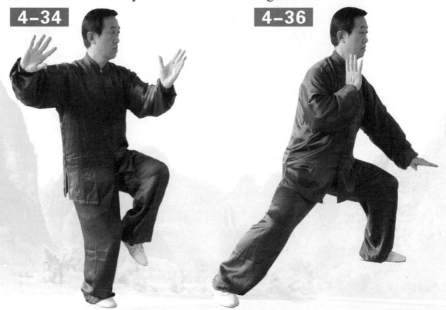

5 As the body turns to the left, transfer the weight on to the left leg and rotate the left arm clockwise. Press the left palm down in a circle (just) below the left knee whilst rotating the arm in a clockwise movement. Push the right palm out and back whilst rotating the arm clockwise and then bring the hand back to be level with the ear rotating the arm counter clockwise with the palm facing into the face. Eyes look forward left. (Figure 4-36)

6 Continue to turn the body to the left and keep the weight on the left leg. Close the left hand to form a Gou-shou - hook, then raise the Gou-shou (five fingers close together to form a hook) to shoulder level in an arc. The right palm pushes to the front of the chest. Eyes look forward. (Figure 4-37)

Key requirements to the movement:
Use the wrist to lead the movement when lifting the left Gou-shou.

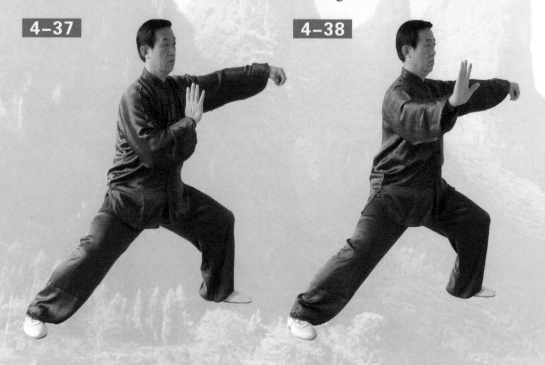

4-37   4-38

7 Turn the body to the right and push the right palm forward, and then to the right in an arc. Keep the shoulders and hips relaxed, with the chest in, knees bent, and waist and elbows sunk down. Eyes look forward. (Figure 4-38)

Key requirements to the movement:
The posture requires an upright, loose and open body with the legs forming an arch shape. The head is erect and the strength is held with mental awareness. Both the arms and feet should be located in a diagonal direction. This is called the Centralized Body Posture. Breathe out during this movement.

Form 8 Brush Knee

1 The body sinks down with relaxed hips and bent knees whilst the left Goushou reverts to a palm. Push both arms down in a circular motion to bring them close together with the left arm rotating counter clockwise and the right arm clockwise. Both arms are located above the left knee with the right palm to the inside of the left forearm. The weight remains on the left leg and the eyes look forward and down. (Figure 4-39)

Key requirements to the movement:
Prior to pushing both arms down, both hands are lifted up in outward circles. As the body sinks down both arms push down in a closing movement as if pushing against water with co-ordinated strength. Breathe in on the rise and out on the sinking phase.

2 Bring both palms up in front of the chest to the centerline with the left palm to the fore and the right palm behind. At the same time transfer the weight to the right leg and withdraw the left foot to the front left of the right foot with the toes touching the floor. Bend both knees and relax the hips. Eyes look directly forward. (Figure 4-40)

Key requirements to the movement:
Transfer the weight to the right leg in a downward circle and draw in the left foot naturally. Breathe in during this movement.

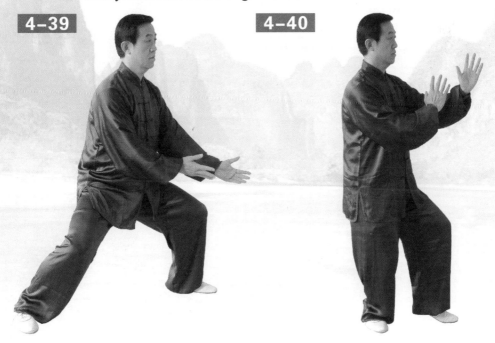

4-39   4-40

Form 9
Stepping to Both Sides (Three Steps Forward)

1 Carry on from the previous movement and turn the body slightly to the right, lift the left foot up with the knee bent. At the same time rotate both arms counter clockwise pulling them down to the right side of the body. Keep all the weight on the right leg with the eyes looking ahead. (Figure 4-41)

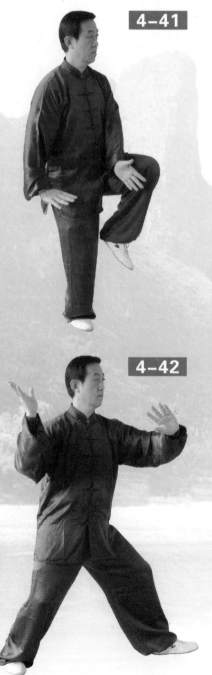

4-41

Key requirements to the movement:
Maintain the ward-off strength whilst pulling down both palms. Form a combined strength between the foot lifting and palms pulling down. Keep the balance stable when standing on the right leg. Breathe out during this movement.

2 Turn the body to the left slightly and the left foot steps out forward with the heel on the floor keeping the toes up. Keep the weight on the right leg and rotate both arms clockwise pushing both palms up and forward. Eyes look forward. (Figure 4-42)

4-42

Key requirements to the movement:
Step out naturally. Co-ordinating the body movement together with pulling both palms down and pushing up. Breathe in while rotating both arms and breathe out as the left foot steps out with the body sinking down.

3 Turn the body to the left more and transfer the weight on to the left leg. Rotate the left arm clockwise further and press it down to the left side of the body. Rotate the right arm counter clockwise and push forward. Lift the right foot up with the knee bent. Eyes look forward. (Figure 4-43).

Key requirements to the movement:
Keep the foot movements stable and rooted.
Step out lightly, flexibly and naturally. For
this movement breathe in at the beginning
and breathe out at the end.

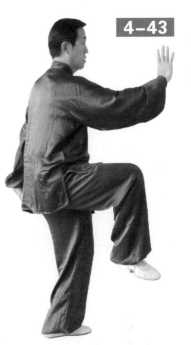

4-43

4 The right foot steps forward and out
with the heel landing on the floor first
with toes lifted up. Keep the weight on
the left leg and turn the body to the left with
the left palm pressing down at the same time
as pushing the right palm forward. Then transfer
the weight forward onto the right leg with the
whole of the foot on the floor. (Figure 4-44).

Key requirements to the movement:
Stepping should be very light and natural,
walk like a cat. The arms should co-ordinate
with the stepping so that the same hand and foot move forwards together.

5 Turn the right toe out then transfer the weight onto the right leg.
Lift the left foot up and step out diagonally forwards. Turn the body
to the right about 90 degrees whilst the left foot steps out and the
right arm rotates counter clockwise with the palm sunk down slightly.
Rotate the left arm counter clockwise pushing it backwards, then rotate
the left arm clockwise and bring the left palm up to the side of the left
ear in an arc,

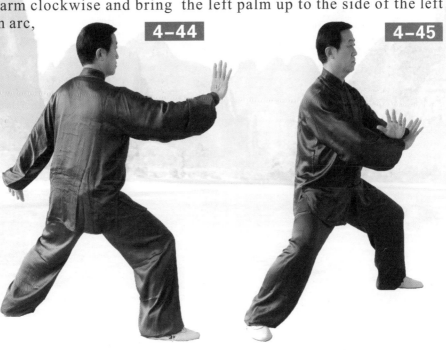

4-44

4-45

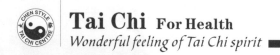

finally the left palm crosses over the right forearm at the front of the chest with the weight on the right leg. Eyes look forward. (Figure 4-45)

Key requirements to the movement:
The body should not rise up whilst stepping out the foot and transferring the weight. Keep the ward off strength in full as both palms cross. Keep the body upright. Breathe in at the beginning and breathe out at the end.

Form 10 Cover hands and Strike with Fist

1 Carry on from the previous movement and turn the body to right slightly with the weight transferring to the left. Both hands press down and separate to the left and right with the left arm rotating clockwise and the right arm rotating counter clockwise. Eyes look forward. (Figure 4-46)

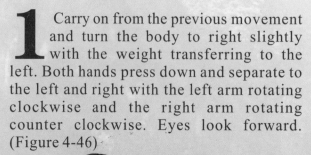

4-46

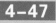

4-47

Key requirements to the movement:
Whilst separating both hands, the body leads the hands. Sinking down is balanced with a flexible circling movement. Breathe in during this movement.

2 Transfer the weight to the right leg with the body turning to the left slightly. Rotate the right arm clockwise and change the right palm to a fist then bring it close to the right waist with the fist facing up. Rotate the left arm counter clockwise and bring the left palm up in front of the chest with the palms facing and the eyes looking forward. (Figure 4-47)

Key requirements to the movement:

Whilst holding the fist to form a 'closing strength', keep your posture upright but sink the body down. Relax the hips and bend the knees slightly. Concentrating the strength on the right leg, prepare the energy to be released. Breathe in during this movement.

3 Transfer the weight on to the left leg by pushing the right foot against the floor with strength and turning the body to the left instantly with the left hip relaxed. At the same time punch the right fist forward with a counter clockwise spiral motion and strike the left elbow backwards simultaneously. The left palm is placed on the left ribs. Eyes look forward over the right fist. (Figure 4-48)

Key requirements to the movement:

Rotating the waist turn the hips whilst the energy is releasing. Punch the right fist forwards instantly with the left elbow striking backward to form a united counter-balanced strength.

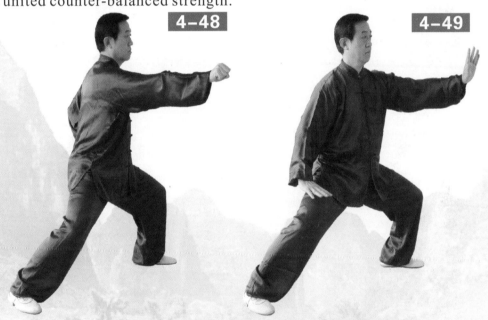

Form 11 High Pat on the Horse

1 Carry on from the previous movement. Keep your weight at the same position, with the body turning right. Change the fist into a palm and pull it back to the side of the right hip in an arc with the right arm rotating counter clockwise slightly and the palm facing down. At the same time push the left palm forward in front of the body with fingers pointing up and the palm facing forward. Eyes look forward. (Figure 4-49)

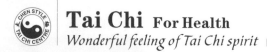
Key requirements to the movement:
Separating of the hands is lead by turning the waist and crotch. The body remains upright and both arms keep hold of the ward off strength, as if the strength fully expands in all directions. During this movement breathe in at the beginning and breathe out at the end.

2 Turn the body to the left with the weight transferring to the right. At the same time turn the right toes in and bring the right palm up in an arc to the right side of the body at the level of the right shoulder with the arm rotating clockwise and the palm facing up. Then bring the right palm to the front of the right shoulder with the arm rotating counter clockwise and the palm facing forward. Whilst moving the right arm, bring the left palm slightly in, with the arm rotating counter clockwise and the palm facing up. The eyes follow the right palm to the end then look over the left palm. (Figure 4-50)

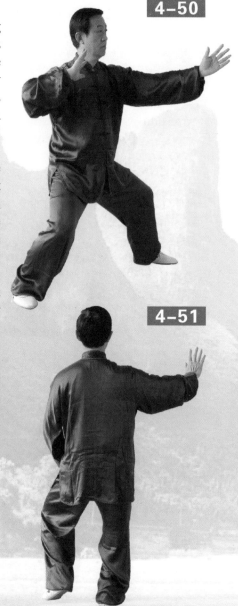

4-50

4-51

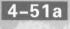

4-51a

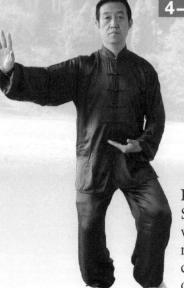

Key requirements to the movement:
Stretch out the chest and relax the hips, whilst bringing the right palm downwards rotating it clockwise. This movement contains the intention of closing while it's open. During this movement breathe in.

3 Turn the body to the left with your weight remaining on the right leg. Withdraw the left foot back to the inside of the right foot in an arc with the toes touching the floor all the time. At the same time push the right palm forward-right in an arc, with the shoulder relaxing and the elbow sinking down. Pull the left palm back to the front of the lower abdomen in an arc with palm facing upwards. Eyes look forward. (Figure 4-51 and 4-51a)

Key requirements to the movement:
Turn the body to the left whilst simultaneously pushing the right palm to the forward-right, with all the body co-ordinated together. During this movement breathe out.

Form 12　Kick with the Left Heel

1 Carry on from the previous movement. Move the left palm out to the forward-left with the arm rotating counter clockwise slightly and the palm facing out, rotate the right arm clockwise with the palm facing out. At the same time transfer the weight to the left leg, whilst lifting your right foot up then move it out to the right side in a large step. (Figure 4-52)

2 Change both hands into fists and keep them softly closed, whilst moving and crossing them in front of your abdomen the fists should face toward the body. At the same time bend the left knee and lift your left foot up with the toes relaxed, hanging under your bottom (groin). Eyes look forward-left. (Figure 4-53 and 4-53a)

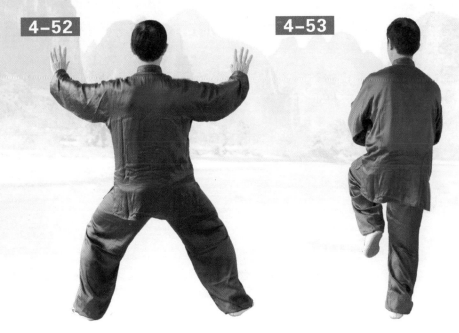

4-52　　4-53

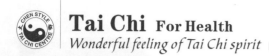

Key requirements to the movement:

Lift the right foot while the body sinks down, with the knee bent and the hips relaxed. The upper body co-operates with the lower body. Both elbows hold ward off strength and are ready to release energy. During this movement breathe in.

3 Use the right leg to support the weight and centre the gravity of the body. Lean the body to the right slightly and kick the left foot out at the level of the lower waist, with your heel. The strength of kicking should come from the waist and hips. At the same time strike both fists to the left and right side of the body and the strength should reach to the surface of the fists. (Figure 4-54)

Key requirements to the movement:

Keep your body balanced on the right leg while both fists and the left foot strike and kick out simultaneously. When the movement closes it is like a hedgehog curling up and when the movement opens, whilst breathing out, it is like a snake striking; an explosion of Qi energy. During this movement breathe out.

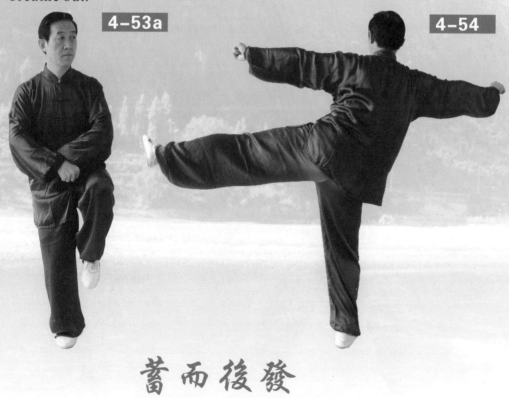

4-53a   4-54

蓄而後發

Form 13 Jade Girl Works at Shuttles

1 Carry on from the previous movement, place the left foot on the floor. Change both fists into palms and then cross them in front of the abdomen with the left arm rotating counter clockwise and the right arm rotating clockwise. (Figure 4-55)

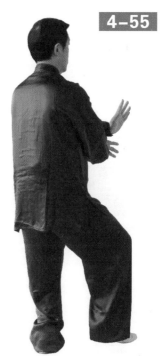
4-55

2 Transfer the weight to the left leg and turn the body to the right. Both palms following the movement of the body, turn to the right and are placed in front of the chest with the fingers pointing up. The right palm is in front of the left palm furthest away from the body with the left palm beside the right elbow. At the same time turn the right knee out and keep the toes on the floor. While turning the body to the right, turn the left toes in. Eyes look forward. (Figure 4-56)

Key requirements to the movement:

While turning the body the waist should be used to direct the shoulders and the shoulders used to direct the elbows, then deliver the ward off strength onto the hands. During this movement breathe in at the beginning and out at the end.

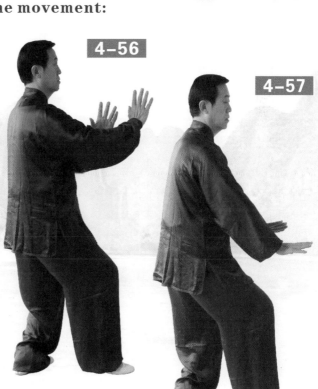
4-56

4-57

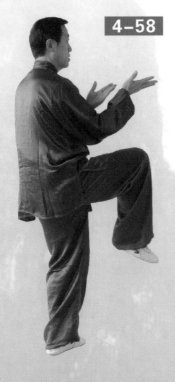

4-58

3 Bend the knees and relax the hips, sink the body down with both hands pressing down and the right arm rotating counter clockwise with the left arm rotating clockwise. Eyes look forward. (Figure 4-57)

Key requirements to the movement:
Do not bend the body while pressing both palms down and sinking the body. During this movement continue breathing out.

4 Both arms lift up with the right arm rotating clockwise and the left arm rotating counter clockwise. At the same time both feet jump up off the ground, lift the right foot before the left. (Figure 4-58)

Key requirements to the movement:
Use the hands to lead the strength and coordinate the whole body whilst jumping lightly. During this movement breathe in.

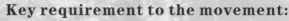

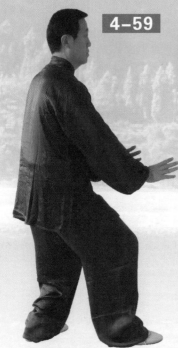

4-59

5 Both feet stamp on the floor with the left foot first then the right. Both hands press down with the right arm rotating counter clockwise and the left arm rotating clockwise. Eyes look forward. (Figure 4-59)

Key requirement to the movement:
Both hands should press down heavily with strength, forming a united movement. Keep the body upright and breathe out.

6 Push both palms up with the right arm rotating clockwise and the left arm rotating counter clockwise. At the same time lift the right foot up with the knee bent. Eyes look forward. (Figure 4-60)

Key requirements to the movement:
Keep the body balanced, rooted and united whilst pushing both palms up and lifting the foot up.

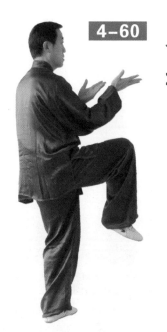

4-60

7 Stand on the left leg and rotate the right leg counter clockwise, slightly, then kick out with the heel. At the same time the right palm pushes out forward with the arm rotating counter clockwise. The left elbow strikes back with the left arm rotating clockwise. Eyes look forward. (Figure 4-61)

Key requirements to the movement:
Release the whole body's strength into the right foot, right palm and left elbow together. Stand firmly on the left leg. During this movement breathe out.

8 The right foot steps forward and lands on the floor, transferring the weight onto the right leg push forward with the right hand. Turn the body to the right slightly and lower the left palm. Eyes look forward. (Figure 4-62)

Key requirements to the movement:
This movement is a transition movement for jumping. The right foot jumps up and kicks forward immediately after landing on the floor. During this movement breathe in at the beginning and out at the end.

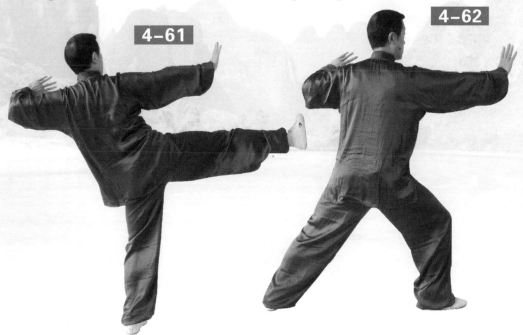

4-61

4-62

9 Push the right foot against the floor and the left foot leap forward onto floor . Turn your body to the right, 180 degrees, and land on the floor on your left foot. At the same time the left palm pushes forward and the right palm moves to the right. The right foot moves across the back of the left foot, keeping the toes on the floor. Eyes look to the left. (Figure 4-63)

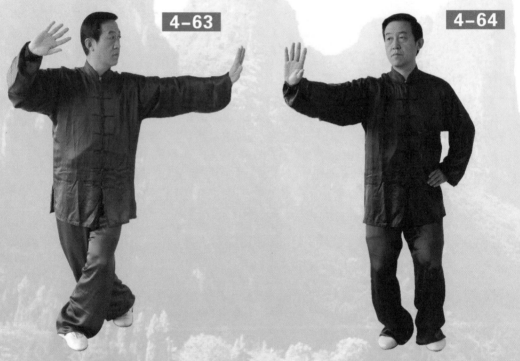

4-63   4-64

Key requirements to the movement:
This is a transition movement. It can be practiced in a continuous motion. It requires landing on the floor lightly and in a balanced fashion.

10 Carry on turning the body to the right for 180 degrees and transfer the weight onto the right leg. The left toes follow the body and turn inward. Both hands pull back to the right with the right arm rotating counter clockwise and the left arm rotating clockwise. The position is shown on the diagram. Eyes look forward-left. (Figure 4-64)

Key requirements to the movement:
Whilst sinking and turning the body both arms hold the ward off strength. During this movement breathe in.

Form 14 Wave Hands

1 Carry on from the previous movement, move the right palm down in an arc to the front of the abdomen with the arm rotating clockwise and the palm facing to the left. At the same time the left palm moves across the front of the body, then pushes to the front of the left shoulder in an arc with the arm rotating clockwise and the palm facing outward-left. Transfer the weight onto the left leg, and then move the right foot to cross behind the left, place the toes on the floor. (Figure 4-65)

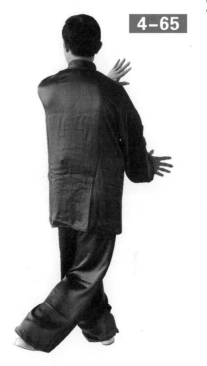

4-65

2 Turn your body to the right slightly and transfer the weight onto the right leg with the whole right foot landing fully onto the floor. Lift your left foot up and move out a step to the left with the heel touching the floor first, keeping the toes lifted up. At the same time move the right hand up, across the front of the body, then push it to the front of the right shoulder with the arm rotating counter clockwise. Push the left palm to the left side, then press down in front of the abdomen in an arc with the arm rotating counter clockwise. Eyes look forward. (Figure 4-66)

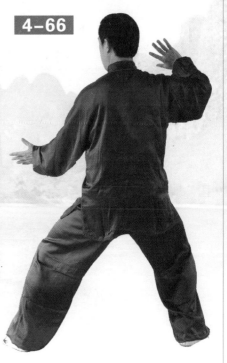

4-66

3 Turn the body to the right slightly and move the right palm down in an arc to the front of the abdomen with the arm rotating clockwise and the palm facing to the left. At the same time the left palm moves across the front of the body then pushes out in front of the left shoulder, but in an arc, with the arm rotating clockwise and the palm facing outwardly left. Transfer your weight onto the left leg, and then move the right foot across and behind the left foot, making sure only the toes land onto the floor. (Figure 4-67)

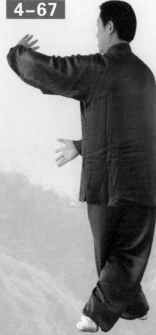

4-67

Key requirements to the movement:

The waist should be the central axis of the movement. Both hands move in an arc in front of the body. Moving one step out and moving one step that crosses behind, together make one whole movement. When crossing behind keep space between the legs and step the toes one pace back. So in order to walk a straight line, to the left, the left foot must move slightly forward during each step subsequent to the first. It is normal to practice four sets but the number of sets can be varied to fit the available space.

Form 15
Turn Body with Double Lotus Kick

1 Carry on from the previous movement by pulling both hands to the back right of the body, with both arms rotating counter clockwise. At the same time turn the body to the right 180 degrees with the body initially turning on the left heel followed by turning on the right heel.

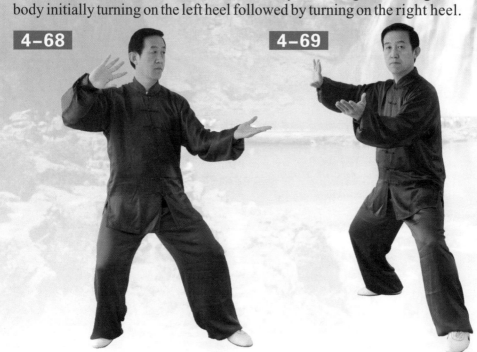

4-68

4-69

The right hand movement ends in front of the middle line of the chest with the palm facing upwards and right. The left hand movement ends in front of the left shoulder with the palm facing up. Eyes look forward-left. (Figure 4-68)

2 Transfer the weight to the right leg and turn the body to the right slightly. Lift the left foot keeping the knee bent then step forward-left with both palms pushing back and to the right. Eyes look forward. (Figure 4-69)

4-70

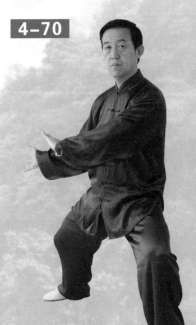

3 Turn the body to the right and transfer the weight to the left leg. Turn both palms back in an arc then press down just beside the right waist. Eyes look forward. (Figure 4-70)

4 Keep the weight on the left leg and lift the right foot up to the left of the body then kick up and swing the foot to the right side of the body. At the same time keep the space between the hands when both palms sweep across to the left and individually strike the outside of the right foot. Eyes look forward. (Figure 4-71)

4-71

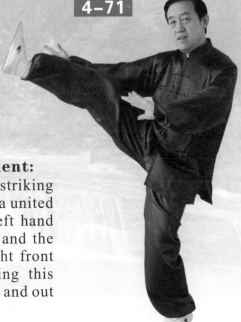

Key requirements to the movement:
The motion of sweeping the foot and striking the palms must be very fast and form a united strength throughout the body. The left hand strikes the foot in front of the body and the right hand strikes the foot at the right front (see illustration Figure 4-71). During this movement breathe in at the beginning and out at the end.

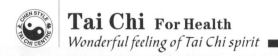

Form 16   Cannon Fist Over Head

1 Carrying on from the previous movement, with the right foot step back one step. Push both hands to the left with both arms rotating counter clockwise. The weight remains on the left leg. Eyes look forward. (Figure 4-72)

Key requirements to the movement:
Keep balance during the foot movements. The hand moves forward along with the foot stepping back should be closed and co-ordinated. During this movement breathe in.

2 Turn your body to the right slightly and transfer your weight onto the right leg. At the same time pull both palms back in front of the right chest and change both palms into fists. Eyes look forward-left. (Figure 4-73)

Key requirements to the movement:
The movement of pulling both palms has to be co-ordinated with the weight transferring and the body turning. Do not bend the waist. During this movement, breathe in first then breathe out.

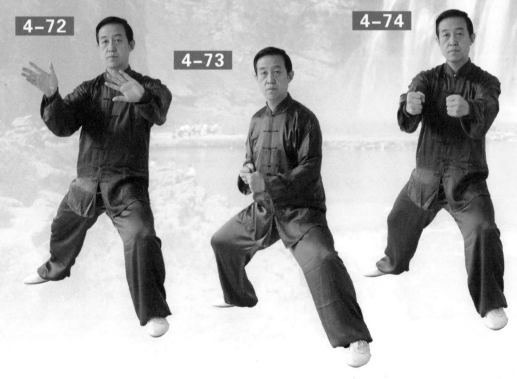

4-72

4-73

4-74

3 Push the right foot against the ground to power the body forward onto the left leg with the body turning to the left. As the body turns to the left both fists fling forward together with the eye of the fist facing upward (see diagram) and both fists facing each other. Eyes look forward. (Figure 4-74)

Key requirements to the movement:
As soon as the mind decides to act, the fists follow instantly realizing energy and shaking powerfully. The movement looks like a golden lion shaking his mane and a powerful tiger jumping down a mountain. The shaking energy is sourced from the waist and hips and should reach the surface of the fists. During this movement breathe out.

Form 17
Buddha's Warrior Attendant Pounds Mortar

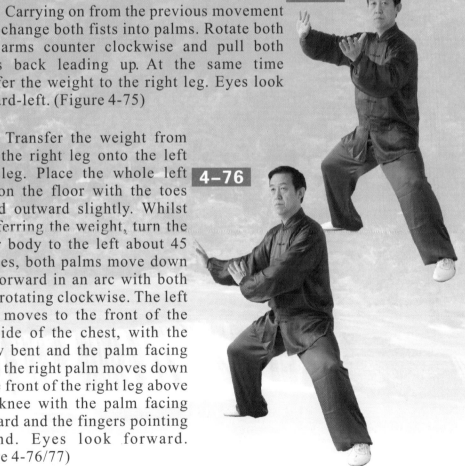

1 Carrying on from the previous movement change both fists into palms. Rotate both arms counter clockwise and pull both palms back leading up. At the same time transfer the weight to the right leg. Eyes look forward-left. (Figure 4-75)

2 Transfer the weight from the right leg onto the left leg. Place the whole left foot on the floor with the toes turned outward slightly. Whilst transferring the weight, turn the upper body to the left about 45 degrees, both palms move down and forward in an arc with both arms rotating clockwise. The left palm moves to the front of the left side of the chest, with the elbow bent and the palm facing down the right palm moves down to the front of the right leg above the knee with the palm facing outward and the fingers pointing behind. Eyes look forward. Figure 4-76/77)

4-75

4-76

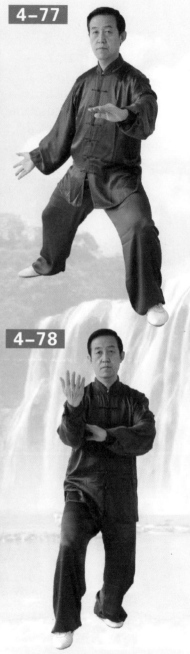

4-77

Key requirements to the movement:
Turning the body, shifting the weight and moving the palms should be co-ordinated. Keep the pelvis down and move the hips forward. The left arm maintains a circular structure and keeps the 'peng' (outward push) strength throughout. Keep the right elbow about 8 to10 centimeters away from the body. The left knee should align vertically above the left ankle. Do not let the knee protrude forward. The right knee is bent and the hips are relaxed. Maintain an arched structure to the legs throughout the movement. Breathe in at the beginning and out at the end of this movement.

3 Keeping the body weight on the left leg, step the right leg forward placing the toes on the ground to create an 'empty stance' (almost no weight on the right foot). At the same time the right hand follows the right leg forward in a rising arc, palm facing upwards in front of the right side of the chest. The fingers of the left hand lightly contact the right forearm. Eyes look forward. (Figure 4-78)

4-78

Key requirements to the movement:
The right foot steps forward with the knees bent, hips relaxed and footwork light, flexible and natural. The movement of the arms co-ordinates with the rise and fall of the body. Breathe in during this movement.

4 The left palm turns upward and sinks down to the front of the lower abdomen. At the same time the right hand forms a fist. Lower the back of the fist into the opened left palm. Eyes look forward. (Figure 4-79)

Key requirements to the movement:
Keep both hands and the abdomen about 8 to 10cm apart, both arms hold a feeling of rounded outward 'peng' strength. The waist sinks down as the fist lowers into the left palm. Breathe out during this movement.

5 Raise the right fist up to shoulder level in front of the body and at the same time, lift the right knee whilst maintaining relaxed hips and a bent left knee. The right toes point naturally downwards and the lower leg is turned slightly inward to a position close to the left knee. Eyes look forward. (Figure 4-80)

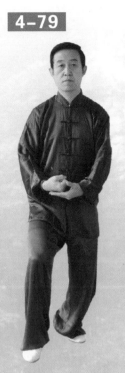

4-79

Key requirements to the movement:
As the right hand and foot rise up, the left side sinks down. (One side of the body is in yin, the other is in yang.) Do not rise up on the supporting leg as the right knee lifts. The internal energy flows down along the body. As the fist rises, the shoulders stay relaxed and the right elbow is dropped down. Breathe in during this movement.

6 Stamp the right foot on the floor about shoulder-width apart from left foot and keep it firmly placed there. At the same time the back of the right fist strikes downward onto the center of the left palm, both arms are bent and maintain a feeling of rounded outward `peng` strength. Eyes look forward. (Figure 4-81)

Key requirements to the movement:
Stamping the foot and pounding the right fist is a co-ordinated power releasing movement. Keep the knees bent and the hips relaxed. The internal energy flows down to the Dantian. Breathe out during this movement.

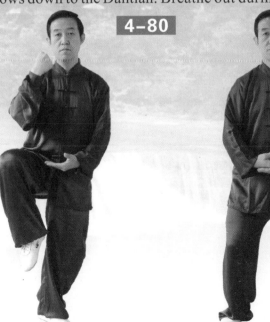

4-80

4-81

Form 18 Finishing Form

1 Carrying on from the previous movement, change the right fist into a palm then split both palms with the body sinking down slightly. Bend the knees and relax the hips. Eyes look forward. (Figure 4-82)

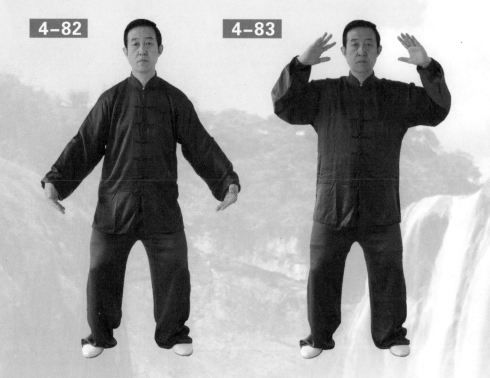

4-82　　4-83

Key requirements to the movement:
While both palms are splitting and the body is sinking down, keep the back upright and do not bend the waist. During this movement breathe in.

2 Carry on to split both hands to both sides of the body and bring them up to shoulder level then turn both the palms over so they are facing downward ending in front of both shoulders. Eyes look forward. (Figure 4-83)

Key requirements to the movement:
While both hands rise up, relax your shoulders and sink the elbow down with the muscles on the chest, abdomen, back and every other part of the body remaining relaxed and sunken. During this movement carry on breathing in.

3 Press both palms down along both sides of the body and end when they are resting at the side of the body. Eyes look forward. (Figure 4-84)

Key requirements to the movement:
While pressing both palms down, breathe out and relax the whole body. The Qi energy will return back to the Dantian (lower abdomen) and the body along with the sprit will become one entity. When you finish the whole series of movements the heart should be quiet and the breathing should be smooth. The movements are continuous -harmonious, with the Qi energy flowing throughout the whole exercise.

4 Return the body slowly to the normal standing position. Eyes look forward and the practice of Taijiquan is completed. (Figure 4-85)

This ends the 18 Short Form

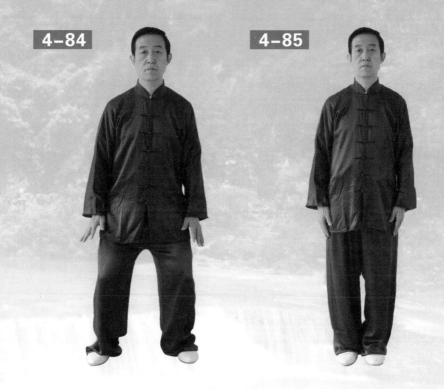

4-84   4-85

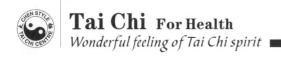

Chapter Five
Views from the West

Whatis Tai Chi? How does Tai Chi relate to your daily life? What are the benefits? Is Tai Chi really good for us or is it just for Chinese people? In this chapter we asked some people from the West to try and answer these questions for you from their own experiences and knowledge.

Section One: A Tai Chi Journey
By Dan Chisholm

In this chapter I will offer a glimpse into the early stages of training, explain the initial phases you will go through and introduce some of the benefits that I have experienced during a decade of training.

Whether old or young, everyone must start at the very beginning. Even the greatest masters were once in the same position that you are now. There are no magic formulas or secret methods to speed up progress, only the requirement of regular study and the guidance from a knowledgeable teacher. Once you begin, you will dive beneath the surface to explore the depths of this fascinating art.

Why Learn Tai Chi?

Most people do not have a clear understanding of Tai Chi. The majority who study see it as a soft and slow exercise with relaxation being the final goal and objective. This concept, whilst being partly correct, is only the first phase of training and barely scratches the surface of a mystical art that extends beyond just physical conditioning. When studying Tai Chi the final objective is to access higher aspects of the self and stimulate latent spiritual abilities using the fusion of body, mind and breath in a form of dynamic meditation.

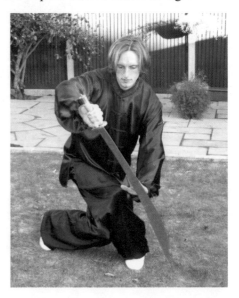

At advanced levels the movements can be performed at any speed. Blending fast and slow, with softness and hardness in a balanced and energetic fluidity that adheres precisely with the ancient Taoist philosophical principles of Yin and Yang. Progress occurs gradually but with patience you will develop a deep understanding of form, movement and internal energy that will generate a wealth of benefits.

Chen Style Tai Chi can be studied all one's life. This complete exercise system contains similar benefits found in both Yoga and Pilates, but includes the additional component of self-defence. Benefits become more profound the longer one studies and includes optimizing health, developing martial skill through the use of internal energy and stimulating spiritual awareness.

Starting Out

In the beginning it is important to learn the basics. Warm-up exercises are studied and begin to promote well-being once simple breathing techniques are employed. Following these initial warm-up routines, silk-reeling energy exercises are introduced. These exercises form the foundation of the longer routines and will help the student to understand the characteristic movements and techniques used. Each exercise is typically undertaken in a fixed position and allows the student to experience a basic level of relaxation and fluidity that will form the basis of their understanding. When learning these techniques you will become immediately aware just how subtle the movements are and how challenging, both physically and mentally, Tai Chi can be. This introduction to Tai Chi is essential and will give students an appreciation of what is involved when studying the more complicated routines.

As a beginner it is important to understand what Tai Chi is, what the fundamental principles are and also what you want to achieve from your practice. If you want good health and a little light exercise, then you need not practice so hard. However, if you want to reach higher levels, then the effort and dedication required will be greater. This is an individual choice and whatever path you take you will accumulate benefits.

I have found through my own teaching that many of my students start practicing Tai Chi as a way to relax and unwind. However, after a short period of study they begin to experience some of the early benefits and then wish to explore a little further.

During this early phase you should begin to develop the ability to relax, both physically and mentally. Movements are performed slowly and softly to draw your attention to areas of stiffness within the body. Once this stiffness is recognised, you can begin to eliminate it and re-educate your body to remain relaxed and to use softness in preference to stiffness.

Initially you will find it difficult to remain relaxed and loose, since stiffness dominates every action you undertake. We are all taught to use stiffness from a young age and unfortunately, this automatic response restricts the circulation of blood and energy. The effect on our circulation by tensing the muscles is like clasping your hands tightly around a hosepipe and squeezing until the flow of water is reduced. This harmful automatic response affects our physical and mental health and must be altered if the maximum benefits from Tai Chi practice are to be achieved. Once our hands (muscles) relax, the water begins to flow naturally again and circulation is restored to normal.

By correcting a student's understanding and letting them experience what relaxation is, they will begin to gain benefits. It is not easy to make this concept clear and even students who have practiced Tai Chi for many years may not fully understand it.

With regular training and careful guidance you will slowly apply this understanding to each movement. Every action will become softer until all movements are made in total relaxation. By heightening your awareness you will be able to apply this principle of relaxation to all areas of your life.

Tai Chi as Meditation

Tai Chi should be thought of as a form of dynamic meditation. Most people think meditation is a practice that involves sitting down with your legs crossed; but meditation should not be confined to just this single activity.

The intricate nature of the Tai Chi routines require the complete co-ordination of mind, body and breath with every action. Through regular repetition these actions become ingrained in the body to allow the mind to focus clearly on their intention and application. Once relaxation and intention are combined, distractive thoughts are removed, internal energy is awakened and a state of meditation is created.

Tai Chi exercises not only teach you to focus the mind but also to create a strong posture - one of the basic requirements for meditation. During seated meditation your body should be strong (but not stiff) to maintain a vertical position of the spine. With correct training your body will gradually become accustomed to holding this posture. Once relaxed, energy will begin to rise up your spine to stimulate the higher energy centres.

Most students will notice the similarity between sitting meditation and the static Tai Chi posture, since no movement occurs. However, students do not seem to associate the flowing movements of the Tai Chi routines in the same way. A student should be able to create the same sensations of energy flow that are experienced during seated meditation in all forms of Tai Chi practice.

At more advanced stages internal energy is stimulated and then circulated. This flow of energy becomes an integral part of the body that initiates movement within the form. This fluidity of action will have a calming meditative influence on the individual practicing but also on those watching - allowing others to benefit from your practice as well.

Early Signs of Progress

As a beginner you will experience a variety of sensations that may excite or confuse you. They are all in fact quite harmless and are just signs to indicate that higher levels are being attained. Some of the early sensations that occur during practice include tingling and sweating, caused by heat generated within the body. These sensations are common and will gradually disappear over time as your body becomes stronger and more accustomed to enhanced circulation of blood and energy.

Of all the techniques learnt in the early stages, the static postures are the most important since they encourage greater internal awareness. By gradually increasing the length of time that you are able to hold these postures, you will begin to produce similar sensations to those indicated below:

1 Relaxing your upper body and sinking at the waist produces a feeling of being strongly rooted to the floor, like being stuck to the floor with glue. This sensation is accompanied by an intense heat in the sole of the foot and is a good indication that blood and energy are circulating freely. These feelings are experienced whilst practicing static postures but are also felt when performing the Tai Chi routines slowly.

2 The standing postures often create a feeling of hot water being poured into the legs. This feeling rises from the feet and begins to fill the thighs. By relaxing, this heat travels up the back and surges over the top of the head and is sometimes combined with a trembling of the thighs. At other times an intense heat swirls and pulsates around the body as it begins to fill the channels with energy, in the same way tributaries are filled following heavy rainfall. These sensations are quite normal and are associated with a feeling of lightness in the upper body and total contentment and connection to your surroundings.

3 Undertaking regular posture training produces strong feelings of energy circulating within, like having a warm river of electricity, or magnetic oil, passing inside your body. This sensation permeates both bone and muscle with a strong vibrating energy. These sensations are astonishing and develop a feeling of internal strength and fluidity of movement that provides great encouragement to continue with your studies.

4 The Tai Chi posture is the simplest to learn, but often the most difficult to perfect. As your body begins to relax from regular training, internal energy begins to circulate freely within. Your skin will become highly sensitive and produces a subtle feeling of warm magnetism surrounding the body, like a "Ready-Brek Glow". This energy strengthens your body and provides protection from the invasion of harmful external pathogens, such as infections and viruses and is one of the important benefits to help strengthen your immune system.

After several years of continued practice your overall ability in the Tai Chi forms and postures will advance. This growth brings with it stronger and more intense feelings that will vary depending upon the health and vitality of each student.

Higher Levels of Development

O nce you become confident and capable in the Tai Chi forms you can begin to apply greater emphasis on the internal aspect of the art.

Through studying Tai Chi you build an awareness of a universal energy that surrounds and permeates us. The training methods help you to access this universal energy like tuning into your favorite radio station and once you receive a strong signal, your movements will begin to flow powerfully.

When the body is soft and flexible, this energy is directed to the extremities in wave-like-pulses, similar to the action of cracking a whip. This wave starts from the feet, travels to the waist and radiates from this central hub, spiraling through the limbs. Unique twisting actions found in Chen Style Tai Chi encourage this energy to travel through the limbs and enhances this flow naturally. This process is only possible once your body is loose and is why so much emphasis is placed on relaxation during the first phase of training.

Once internal energy flow is experienced, the martial application behind the movements becomes clearer. This energy appears gradually and enhances the momentum and fluidity of every action performed. It will take a while for you to reach this level of understanding but it is worth every ounce of practice. As you approach this stage in your training you will begin to see the usefulness of Tai Chi and its effectiveness in a self-defence situation.

During this phase of training your state of mind will play a vital role in your progress. You must first develop the belief that you are capable of performing the movements and with this confidence the seed of intention is sown. If nurtured, it will grow to have a profound influence, not just on your movement, but also in all aspects of your life. Tai Chi promotes a positive outlook and encourages an enthusiasm for life that opens the door for you to explore the furthest reaches of your potential. This outlook will reflect in your behavior towards others and reinforces the feeling of being connected, not isolated from the world you live in.

Benefits from Higher Stages of Practice

The benefits gained during this stage of practice are due to increased levels of energy that circulate through your body's energetic pathways. Relaxation allows this energy to flow and once abundant, is drawn up the spine as a river of vibrating energy, like rising steam. This condensed vapour nourishes your kidneys on its journey to the higher energy centres of the brain before descending vertically down the front of the body, cascading through the throat and chest until it reaches your dantian (abdominal area), where it is drawn into another circuit.

This transportation system occurs in the same way that water from the ocean evaporates, traveling in the form of clouds and cascading as rain on the earth, until eventually returning back to the sea again by means of streams and rivers. This action will continue to nourish your whole body, as long as your energy remains strong and the body and mind are relaxed and calm.

Tai Chi was developed with a profound understanding of these energetic pathways. Through unique spiraling actions found in Chen Style Tai Chi these pathways are freed from blockages to allow energy and fluid to flow smoothly. Once this occurs, your body returns to its original state of optimum health.

Every movement you undertake reinforces the opening and clearing of these pathways, in the same way a Chinese doctor would aim to do using Acupuncture or Tui Na massage. Tai Chi exercises have been used for centuries as an effective supplement to Chinese Medicine, used to strengthen the body and to promote a long and healthy life.

In Conclusion

One should always be aware that Tai Chi is in the body, not in the mind. You may read and theorize about it, but a true understanding only comes from continued practice. Just keep reminding yourself of the old saying "practice makes perfect".

I am very fortunate to have begun my own journey under the guidance of two exceptional teachers, Master Liming Yue and Grandmaster Chen Zhenglei. This level of instruction has given me a deeper understanding of this incredible art and I will be forever grateful for all that I have been taught. Even after a decade of training, I am still enthusiastic and excited in what lies ahead, always aware just how much there is still to learn.

Section Two
Tui Na Chinese Massage and Chen Style Taijiquan
By Nick Taylor

What do Tui Na Chinese massage and Taijiquan have in common? They have their origins rooted in Traditional Chinese Medicine, and both utilize similar techniques for improving health, fitness and longevity. This chapter is an introduction to Tui Na, a comparison of some of the techniques employed within both disciplines, and an explanation of the health benefits arising from these remarkable skills.

The Discovery

From my early days of training with Master Liming Yue, I still recall the powerful and energetic feelings I enjoyed after each Taijiquan class. I felt more energized, calm, relaxed and happy, even if it was hard work. These benefits came from simple, effective exercises, created hundreds of years ago in China. Throughout a decade of training in Taijiquan, my interest in Chinese culture, especially the health and medical aspects, deepened. It was during this period that I heard about something called Tai Chi massage from Master Liming Yue and other Taijiquan masters. Correctly called Tui Na, my first Tai Chi massage was amazing, great movements of Qi energy flowed up and down my spine, throughout my back, and I felt calm and more relaxed. These sensations I recognized as similar to those that I had experienced during my Taijiquan practice. This discovery encouraged me to train in Tui Na Chinese massage, and to eventual qualification as a Tui Na Master Practitioner.

Tui Na Chinese Massage

Tui Na (pronounced twee nah) simply means to push and grasp. Powerful and effective, Tui Na is used to remedy training injuries, heal the body, improve health by balancing Qi energy and stimulate the immune system. For many high level practitioners of Taijiquan, the use of Tui Na is also important in support of their training routine. Tui Na is a branch of Chinese medicine that is guided by the theories of Traditional Chinese Medicine and is equal in importance to acupuncture and herbal treatment for the maintenance of good health, balance and harmony. Traditional Chinese Medicine is founded on the concepts of treating the body as an integrated whole, the theory of Yin and Yang, and understanding the meridians through which Qi energy flows.

An important feature of Tui Na is that the practitioner stands in a relaxed, stable posture. This enhances the benefits gained from the four main features of Tui Na techniques, which are rhythm, frequency, duration and strength. Adopting the correct posture also helps the practitioner enter into a quiescent state, and by relaxing the body, enables Qi energy to descend to the dantien. In this state of mind, combined with regular, even breathing, the practitioner guides their Qi energy and the power of the whole body into the hands, further empowering the treatment. These skills can be developed and greatly enhanced through the practice and study of Chen Style Taijiquan.

The Healing Effects of Tui Na Chinese Massage

T he curative qualities and medical benefits of Tui Na Chinese massage can be applied to injuries, and acute or chronic conditions, both physical and emotional. Tui Na successfully treats stress, migraine, headache, insomnia, tension and restlessness. It is effective in treating repetitive strain injuries such as tenosynovitis, bursitis, carpal tunnel syndrome, tennis elbow and golfers elbow. Tui Na relieves the pain of cervical spondylosis, acute

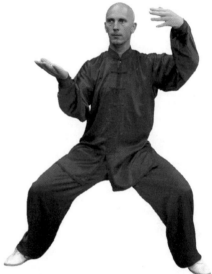

lumbar strain, prolapsed intervertebral lumbar disc (slipped disc), stiff neck, whiplash injury and sacro-iliac joint problems. Rheumatoid arthritis, spinal osteoarthritis, facial paralysis, and torticollis also respond well to Tui Na. Tui Na works well in the treatment of sports injuries. As a result of the improved flow of Qi energy stimulated by the massage techniques, the healing process is enhanced, especially for the inert connective tissues such as tendons, ligaments and cartilage.

The development of unhindered, smooth flowing Qi energy through Tui Na Chinese massage is appropriate for healing specific medical conditions and for self-maintenance by Taijiquan practitioners. It has an ability to improve physical performance, aids all sports people and creates a healthier, more active life for friends and family. The physical benefits of Tui Na treatments are enjoyable for those in need of healing and pain release, and also for improving the general quality of life.

Tui Na Techniques and Chen Style Taijiquan

T he Tui Na manipulations discussed here are some of the many standard technical maneuvers used for treating injuries, improving health and balancing Qi. The Tai Chi forms movement Cover Fist and Punch, prepares for, and then releases energy. The right fist strikes out forwards, and at the same time the left elbow strikes backwards. This form contains similar movement properties as the Tui Na manipulations Ban, to pull, and Bashen, to pull/extend. Here, the main principle is a firm pull by the Tui Na practitioner at both ends of a joint, in opposite directions. This effect can also be achieved during many of the other powerful, energy release, Fa Jing movements characteristic of Chen Style Taijiquan. The medical benefits achieved from this Tai Chi strike/Tui Na manipulation include a reduction in articular disturbances. These are partial dislocations of the shoulder joint, which can become fixed, causing osteoarthritis and a loss of articular surface on the head of the humerus. Articular adhesion (common cause of frozen shoulder) can also be corrected, and lubrication of the joints improved. The effects of physical deformities are rectified and the normal range of motion restored to joints. Other health benefits include the treatment and repair of injured soft tissues, and the alleviation of nerve compression. Nerve compression can cause problems such as numbness and tingling in the hands, arms, legs and feet. Further advantage gained from this type of Tai Chi strike/Tui Na manipulation is a widening of the joint spaces, allowing more Qi energy to flow through, fill the joint and clear energetic blockages. This can also enhance joint lubrication, reduce inflammation and help to improve cartilage protection. In addition the tendons are stretched, helping to improve their strength and flexibility.

The Chen Style Tai Chi Warm Up exercises which include circling the waist, knee exercises, elbow circling around the shoulder, circling the head, arm circling around the elbow, and wrist rotation contain similar movement properties as the Tui Na manipulation Yao, to rotate. The massage techniques flex, extend and rotate the body within the normal range of movement. The medical benefits available from both approaches include improving the function of the joints, reducing stiffness and soreness, and treating articular adhesion. Other effective improvements to health that can be achieved apply to acute sports injuries, such as muscle strain involving myofascial damage and limited muscle fibre injury, repetitive strain injury, tendinitis, tennis elbow, golfers elbow and also osteo-arthritis and rheumatoid arthritis. These Chen Style Taijiquan exercises and Tui Na manipulations also prepare the joints of the body for relaxing and opening up, creating the situation in which joint spaces can increase, allowing for improved Qi energy flow. The side to side twist of the upper body in the Warm Up exercises also contains similar attributes as the Tui Na shoulder to hip spinal twist manipulation, which is used for treating chronic lower lumbar pain and sciatica.

In general, the spiraling and circular movements characteristic of Chen Style Taijiquan cause the arms and shoulder joints to move in flexion/extension, abduction/adduction and in circumduction. In turn, the musculature of the upper arm, shoulder, upper back and scapula continuously stretch and relax. The scapula, suspended in a network of muscles, tendons and ligaments can be elevated, depressed, moved laterally or medially and rotated towards or away from the spine. All of these complex movements greatly assist in soothing and releasing upper back tension, allowing for a normalization in the flow of Qi energy, and improving blood circulation. Also enhanced is the flow of lymph fluid, which transports essential vitamins to the blood, facilitates immune responses and drains excess interstitial fluid from tissue spaces. During the course of a Tui Na shoulder and upper back treatment, similar health benefits are achieved, with the addition of the wonderful feelings of increased energy typically experienced after a Tui Na treatment.

The spiraling and circular actions that are key components of Chen Style Taijiquan and Silk Reeling exercises contain within them the self-defence elements called Peng (ward off), Lu (roll back), Ji (squeeze) and An (press). In combination, the arm and hand movements display similar properties as the Tui Na manipulation Gung Fa. In the manipulation Gung Fa, also called Chinese rolling, the back of the hand rolls backward and forwards repetitively, in a smooth rhythmic manner. The effectiveness of this manipulation is achieved through the frequency of repetition, and the integrated and relaxed use of the whole body to deliver different levels of power. Starting at the shoulder, the rolling movement continues through the upper arm, into the elbow, is amplified by the forearm, which gently rotates inward and outward, and then transferred through rotation and flexion of the wrist to the hand. The medical health benefits gained from either the Tai Chi or Tui Na approach include a relaxation of the muscles and tendons, helping to reduce and eliminate the painful effects of repetitive strain injuries. In particular, Gung Fa helps to increase the flow of Qi energy, which helps to warm the meridians and dispel dampness.

The dynamic, flowing movement of the Warm Up exercises, Tai Chi forms and Silk Reeling exercises improve blood circulation and Qi energy flow. The Tui Na manipulations Yao, (rotate), Gung Fa, (rolling), Pai, (pat), Dou, (shake) Tui, (push) Na, (grasp), and Ca, (rub), all play a part in regulating and balancing the flow of Qi energy and blood. The act of doing some form of exercise increases the heart rate and blood flow. In Traditional Chinese Medicine, blood and Qi are considered interdependent. They have a unique relationship whereby Qi creates and promotes blood circulation and is said to be the commander of the blood. Qi receives its nourishment and nutrition from blood.

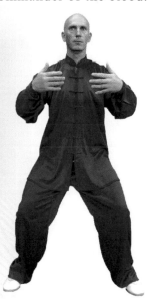

Blood is said to be the mother of Qi. Qi invigorates blood and Qi deficiency can result in blood stagnation or some form of blood deficiency. Blood is Yin and Qi is Yang. In partnership or individually, Tai Chi and Tui Na create an improvement in Qi and blood circulation, enabling the whole body to fulfil its metabolic activities. Regular Taijiquan practice can also improve the condition known as Raynauds Disease. This disease affects the blood supply to the fingers and toes, with accompanying skin colour changes, coldness and numbness. It is believed that poor circulation and emotions such as stress and anxiety contribute to this disease. Tui Na can also ameliorate this condition through the massage techniques and the accompanying boost to the immune system typical after a treatment.

Individual Taijiquan practice strengthens and harmonizes the body, helping to protect it from disease and restore good health. A Tui Na practitioner enables the individual to achieve good health, eliminate disease and maintain homeostasis. Tui Na Chinese massage is treatment specific, boosts the immune system and is a holistic method of natural healthcare. This baton of good health is then sustained and improved upon by regular Taijiquan practice. Both methods use the same Qi energy principle discovered by the ancients, thousands of years ago. In my experience as a Taijiquan Instructor and Tui Na Practitioner I see the two disciplines as being vital strands in the quest for a healthy life, woven from the same braid of knowledge.

For further reading and reference, the following books will be useful to the reader: *The Web That Has No Weaver* by Ted J. Kaptchuk; *Fundamentals of Chinese Medicine* by Nigel Wiseman & Andrew Ellis; *Chinese Tui Na Massage* by Xu, Xiangcai; *Chinese Tuina Therapy* by Wang Fu; *The Seirin Pictorial Atlas of Acupuncture* by Yu-Lin Lian.

Section Three
Managing Stress with Tai Chi
By Bill Wilkinson

What is stress?

The Health and Safety Executive (HSE) defines stress as "the adverse reaction people have to excessive pressure or other types of demands placed on them".

Pressure is part and parcel of daily life and helps to keep us motivated both in our work and social lives. But excessive pressure can lead to stress that undermines performance, is costly to employers and can make people ill.

Why do we need to tackle stress?
HSE commissioned research has indicated that:

About half a million people in the UK experience work-related stress at a level they believe is making them ill.

Up to 5 million people in the UK feel "very" or "extremely" stressed by their work; and a total of 12.8 million days were lost to stress, depression and anxiety in 2003/4.

HSE key messages on stress:

HSE is working with businesses to enable them to manage work related stress more effectively.

Work related stress is a serious problem. Tackling it effectively can lead to significant benefits for organizations. There are practical things that organizations can do to prevent and control work related stress. Stress is a management issue which managers can help to resolve.

Everyday an estimated 270,00 employees are absent from work because of work related stress. However, only 13% of companies have implemented schemes to combat it. Stress at work is still not taken seriously despite its being one of the biggest problems facing employers and employees in the workplace today. Despite the cost to the "bottom line" in terms of increased cost and lost revenue in productivity, companies in the UK are doing little to deal with this growing threat.

We will all have suffered from some form of stress in our working lives, whether knowing it or not. In these hectic times, stress isn't limited to the office. HSE also commissioned some research which identified that those working in the education sector, including non-teaching staff, are some of the most likely to be exposed to psychosocial hazards that can lead to work related stress. Furthermore, 42% of teachers and 23% of those in education and welfare roles report high levels of stress.

Additionally, there have been many studies conducted on the effects of stress on schoolchildren. Some research has even suggested that over 90% of schoolchildren feel stressed at school, the main reason often cited is doing well at school. In the year April 1, 2003 to March 31, 2004, more than 900 children and young people called Child-Line, the free 24 hour help-line, about the stress caused by their exams - up from just over 600 in the previous 12 months.

If the Government's own research through the HSE has estimated that 1 in 5 people are stressed at work, then we have a significant potential health problem looming in the UK. The Revitalizing Health and Safety Strategy was launched jointly by the Government and the Health and Safety Commission on 7 June 2000. It is a 10 year strategy seeking to make significant improvements in workplace health and safety by setting targets for reducing incidences of work related ill-health and working days lost caused by injury and ill-health.

The targets to meet by 2010 relating to work-related stress include:

A 20% reduction in the incidence of work-related ill health and a 30% reduction in the number of work days lost due to work-related ill health. That people not working due to ill health or disability are given opportunities for rehabilitation back into work or offered opportunities to prepare for and find employment.

From an employers point of view, this focus by the government on improving the incidences of work related stress should be seen as a positive step. An Employee Well Being programme in the workplace could have a significant effect on the profitability of a company by:

Reducing absence rates through stress management techniques which will reduce costs by spending less on other employees having to work overtime to cover the absentee.

Reducing turnover as employees are more motivated to stay with a caring employer will reduce the costs of recruitment, selection and training.

Improving productivity through more staff being at work at any one time.

These three positive outcomes contribute to a reduction in costs and an increase in income, resulting in an improved profit line for a company. However, companies need to invest time and money in looking for a solution that will help their employees.

So what is stress and what problems both mental and physical can develop? The body has an inbuilt physical response to stressful situations. Faced with pressure, challenge or danger, we need to react quickly, and our bodies release hormones such as cortisol and adrenaline to help us do this. These hormones are part of the "fight or flight" response and affect the metabolic rate, heart rate and blood pressure, resulting in a heightened - or stressed - state that prepares the body for optimum performance in dealing with a stressful situation.

Very often, modern stresses do not call for either fight or flight. Nevertheless, the same stressing hormones are released as part of the reaction and this natural reaction to challenge or danger, instead of helping, can damage health and reduce the ability to cope.

In the wake of the growing number of individuals experiencing stress at a potentially problematic level at home and in the work place, stress counselors and stress management companies are mushrooming. They promote their solutions to companies to help them manage this deteriorating situation.

Most of us at some time feel the pressures of modern life. We exercise a lot less than our parents and grandparents. Trying to achieve a reasonable work/home balance can often prove very challenging. Most of the time we manage to "cope" with the situations we are in. However, for some people it has become so difficult that they look for some respite in drink or even drugs. All of these things are contributing to an increasingly unhealthy lifestyle, which makes us less able to deal with stress on a physical as well as an emotional level.

So how can Tai Chi help?

From my own personal experience, I have found that Tai Chi has helped me to cope with a full time, very demanding, professional job working for one of the UK's leading banks. My wife (who also has a very demanding job as a Director) and I have raised two daughters so we are both fully aware of the stresses that people are being confronted with on a day-to-day basis.

We both took up Tai Chi at the same time over five years ago, firstly with Steve Burton in Accrington and then Master Liming Yue in Manchester Tai Chi Centre. I have an old injury to my back and my physiotherapist recommended Tai Chi for its health promoting benefits. Over this period, we have both found that the regular practice of Tai Chi and particularly Qigong has enabled us to relax both physically and emotionally. The meditative practices of Qigong provide a very welcome opportunity to take some time out and try to understand the tensions and stresses that exist in our bodies.

According to Master Liming Yue, Tai Chi can have a dramatic effect on people's health. When practicing Tai Chi, the practitioner's consciousness, breathing and actions are all closely connected. Tai Chi exercises stimulate both blood circulation and the internal organs, as well as improving strength and muscle control. Tai Chi helps to improve health, co-ordination and posture along with enhancements to general fitness and weight loss. It stimulates the body and calms the mind, resulting in a balanced outlook and an overall improved sense of well being.

It helps mind and body to relax. I used to think that I was able to relax but since I started practicing Tai Chi, I soon realized that my body was in a permanent state of tension caused by the conscious and subconscious stresses of everyday life. Left unattended these stresses can cause long-term damage and ill health, as previously discussed.

Practicing Tai Chi has not prevented stress happening in my life whether at work or at home. It is not a panacea for all personal issues. What it can do is improve physical, mental and spiritual health and well-being. In helping to relax body and mind, it has put me in a better position to cope with the demands that are being placed on my body. It helps maintain my body in a better condition, thus helping the body to reduce the risks of more permanent damage that stress can cause. Stress is a major cause of illness and ill health. It is also a significant reason for ill health in the work place. So much so that companies in the UK are looking for some solutions to reduce the incidences of absence and to meet the Governments

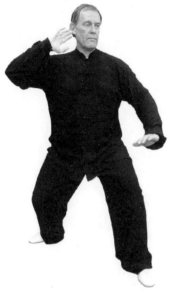

challenging targets. Tai Chi is ideal for the workplace as it is so simple to incorporate. It is surprising that more companies have not instituted this sensible programme for keeping their employees fit. On a practical note, there is no need for expensive gymnasiums, equipment, showers or sportswear. It can be practiced on your own in the workplace or as part of an organized class during the working day.

Equally, in the school playground, whether as a teacher, assistant or a pupil, Tai Chi exercise can have a very positive effect on improving the behaviour of school-children. Teachers at a primary school in Wiltshire introduced Tai Chi classes in 2000 to encourage children to concentrate on their lessons. 48 pupils at a Church of England school took part in exercise sessions every morning before classes started. BBC news reported a teacher as saying, " After doing their Tai Chi the children come into the classroom and it really quietens them down - they are more prepared for their work and it creates a better atmosphere in the school."

Whether at work or in school, regular practice of Tai Chi can help your body to minimize the longer term damaging effects that stress can cause. Solutions that help companies and schools deal with the human and financial costs involved in stress related illness or activity would be welcomed. At an individual level, regular practice may also help put some of the issues or problems that you are facing into perspective by enabling you to relax more deeply both physically and mentally.

Acknowledgments:

Health and Safety Executive: Work-related stress; Health and Safety Executive's research in "The Scale of Occupational Stress", CRR 311/2000; Teacher Support Network: BBC News Archive- Education-18/9/2000

Section Four
Tai Chi & Qigong for the Elderly
By Sifu Steven Burton

There are many millions of people of all ages who practice Tai Chi and Qigong around the world. These people find that the health benefits they gain last everyday throughout their life.

The Western perception of Chinese people practicing in the parks early morning is almost mystical yet this wonderful art is accessible to each and every one of us.

You can perform Tai Chi well into your eighties and nineties and receive its life sustaining health care benefits. Could the same be said for jogging, weight lifting, and aerobics? Due to the harsh impact nature of jogging and many other exercises, during the long term the joints suffer whereas with Tai Chi and Qigong your physical and mental health is maintained and improved.

To illustrate all the benefits would take an encyclopedia, but I will focus on some of the key benefits that can be derived from regular practice.

Benefits include:

1. Prevention or therapy of arthritic pain.
2. Improved balance
3. Reduced stress levels
4. Improved blood circulation and general cardiovascular system
5. More efficient breathing
6. Maintenance and improvement in co-ordination
7. Strengthening of the immune system
8. Increased mobility and flexibility

Pain free movement:

When practicing the slow rhythmical movements of Tai Chi all the joints of the body are worked gently through their natural range of motion. It is a well known fact that one must keep joints mobile to ease or prevent arthritic pain. Many physiotherapists would give gentle exercises to mobilize the joints and therefore I see Tai Chi as being a kind of D.I.Y physiotherapy. In medical terms the movements of Tai Chi will cause the bodies synovia membranes to produce the lubricant (synovia fluid) within the joints and thus allow the joints to "glide" more easily.

Balance for life:

A study at Emory University shows significant decrease in the incidents of falling after practicing the ancient art of Tai Chi.

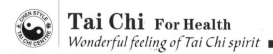

The Emory study looked at seven therapeutic benefits for Tai Chi:

1. Continuous movement.

2. Small to large degrees of motion depending on the individual.

3. Flexed knees with distinct weight shifts between legs.

4. Straightening and extending head and trunk for less 'flexed' posture. Attention developed to prevent leaning of trunk or protrusion of the sacrum.

5. Trunk and head rotates as a unit during circular movements that emphasize rotation. Eyes follow movement, promoting head and trunk rotation through eye centering and eye movements.

6. Asymmetrical and diagonal arm and leg movements promote arm swing and rotation around the waist axis.

7. Unilateral weight bearing with constant shifting to and from right and left legs to build strength for unilateral weight bearing and improve unilateral balance through knowledge of one's balance limitations and practice of movements within those limitations.

The core principles of Tai Chi and Qigong are posture alignment controlled movement. The very nature of Tai Chi exercise is to work on core stability and balance. Tai Chi practice makes people feel more confident about movement and posture through practice and therefore as quite a number of falls are caused by lack of confidence this is one way falls are prevented as ones confidence improves.

The power of breath:

One of the most essential ingredients for performing at your best is to understand the proper and most efficient way to breathe. Whatever you do from walking to more vigorous activities, proper breathing is essential for success. Tai Chi and Qigong incorporates this necessary ingredient through full deep abdominal breathing and knowing when to inhale and exhale for each movement. Unfortunately, most people do not know how to breath correctly.

Look at babies for the correct method of breathing, babies are not taught how to breathe at birth, it just happens. Their little bellies are pumping away giving them optimal energy. Their arms and legs move freely with ease. As we get older many people tend to restrict their breathing. People begin shallow breathing from their chests only. This limited kind of breathing puts a limit to our bodies natural potential. Breath is life! The value of deep abdominal breathing as we practice in Tai Chi, is essential for increasing your quality of life more than you would believe.

Through improved breathing and gentle movement comes stimulation of the circulation and as we breath the body becomes energized due to the increase in oxygen to the lungs and continuing the journey, through to every cell of our bodies.

As our blood carries oxygen around our bodies and through deep Qigong breathing our lungs are working more efficiently it is easy to see that this alone justifies why we should practice Tai Chi. Tai Chi nourishes our bodies and WILL improve your life if practiced regularly.

Correct diaphragmatic breathing can also improve back pain due to the fact that the diaphragm has connective tissue to the lumbar spine and correct breathing can cause one to relax the muscles in the back.

Due to the very nature of relaxed controlled breathing the practitioner will find themselves in a state of both mental and physical relaxation which in turn can help to regulate blood pressure as stress levels reduce. Breath is Life !

In fact the rhythmical movement of the diaphragm and abdominal muscles during correct breathing could be said to massage the internal organs such as the intestines liver, stomach, etc. & therefore keep the internal organs healthy.

The amazing immune system:

Our bodies naturally have an amazing ability to regenerate tissue if damaged and to combat illness of many sorts. Unfortunately, due to today's society and dietary trends, our immune system tends not to work as efficiently as it can.

During Qigong and Tai Chi practice one of the requirements of training is that the tip of the tongue is placed gently to the roof of the mouth. There are many physical and meta-physical benefits of doing so. The main one that I will focus on is the fact that by placing the tongue thus causes the saliva production to increase. Within saliva there is an enzyme called 'amylase' which is responsible for the first stages of digestion. This is one of the reasons why it is recommended to thoroughly chew food before swallowing it, as the amylase mixes with the food and begins the digestion process. A healthy digestive system means a strong immune system.

Medisch Dossier (volume 6, number 7), a Dutch medical newsletter, reports on a study where a group of older men and women (average age of 70) practiced Tai Chi three days a week for 45 minutes. After fifteen weeks they not only felt much more healthy, but had twice the number of immune cells (called T-cells) which are specially equipped to knock out the virus that causes shingles and also many other viruses.

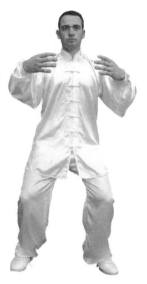

Jim Plant

Tai Chi Practitioner (Darwen Falls prevention classes) " I began Tai Chi under the tuition of Steven Burton about 1 year ago. I was prompted by the Health and Fitness development team of Blackburn with Darwen Borough Council to try Tai Chi as they believed that it would help improve my mobility and balance.

I have always been active and in my youth was a very sporty person, but I have never come across a more concise series of exercises as Tai Chi. The exercises work both the physical external muscles and joints as well as working all the internal organs through the breathing techniques. All the movements are gentle and there is no stress to any joints. My health has improved so much. I find Tai Chi truly amazing! "

The list of benefits are seemingly endless but the most important thing is to enjoy your journey into the study of this fascinating art.

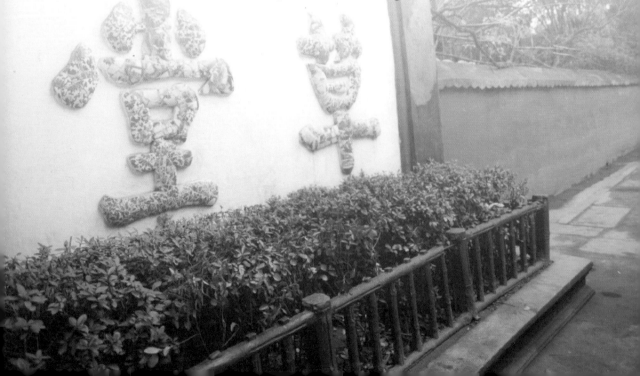

Section Five
Traditional Chinese Medicine & Tai Chi
Promoting mental, physical and spiritual health
By Professor Shulan Tang
Founder of Shulan College of Chinese Medicine.
Academic Executive of ATCM UK.
Fellow Member of Registrar of Chinese Herbal Medicine, UK.
Member of the British Acupuncture Council, UK.

Introduction

I have been practicing Chinese medicine in England since 1991. The majority of my patients are westerners, suffering mainly from depression, anxiety and low energy, especially during the long cold winters here. Along with acupuncture and Chinese herbal medicine, I believe Tai Chi is excellent for treating physical excesses as well as mental and emotional problems. For pure relaxation it has no equal.

The close links between Traditional Chinese Medicine (TCM) and Tai Chi Chuan have long been familiar to the Chinese - both are based on the core value of balance and harmony, and the belief that balance is essential for a long and healthy life, physically, mentally and emotionally. This balance can best be summed up by the Yin-Yang concept.

The main foundation for TCM is that of universal energy, or Qi (pronounced as chee), which surrounds us and is necessary for all living things, whether plants, animals or humans. Qi is considered positive and negative, dynamic and static, passive and aggressive, Yin and Yang - complementary opposing forces. In the human body, this energy circulates along channels known as meridians. There are points along these channels which can affect the flow of Qi, thus directly altering the body's essential balance and harmony. If certain blockages or imbalances occur, this can result in illness. TCM assumes that a balance between Yin and Yang is the key to health.

There are many ways to influence the flow of yin and yang: TCM is one way, by prescribing herbs to treat certain excesses or deficiencies in the patients constitution; acupuncture is another, involving the manipulation of certain points on the meridians to stimulate Qi flow; and Tai Chi can also act to attract and circulate Qi

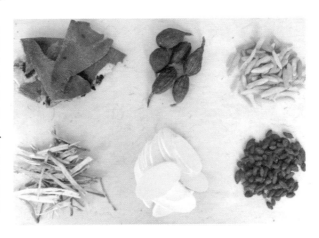

through the body in a steady way, rectifying any imbalances through gentle exercise. When your body is ready, more vigorous exercises will produce even greater benefits.

The medical classic of the Yellow Emperor, produced over two thousand years ago, states clearly that the concept of Yin-Yang is at the heart of everything, including life and death, and this belief is the basis for TCM treatment as well as Tai Chi forms of shadow boxing, pushing movements offset with pulling, left movements with right, forwards with backwards.

What makes Tai Chi special?

There are four main features of Tai Chi: it is gentle and relaxing, a non-impact activity suitable for all ages and nearly all conditions of health; it is fluid and uniform in movement - there are no sudden stops and starts as in many sports; it is circular and cyclical, the forms bringing you through a series of smooth movements to finish back where you started; and it is integrated and complete, gently working the whole body, exercising the mind and powers of concentration and breathing techniques, while working on the inner organs at the same time.

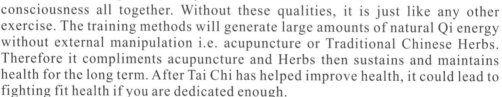

It is the most popular type of exercise that uniquely combines breathing, mind, body movements and consciousness all together. Without these qualities, it is just like any other exercise. The training methods will generate large amounts of natural Qi energy without external manipulation i.e. acupuncture or Traditional Chinese Herbs. Therefore it compliments acupuncture and Herbs then sustains and maintains health for the long term. After Tai Chi has helped improve health, it could lead to fighting fit health if you are dedicated enough.

Health benefits of practicing Tai Chi

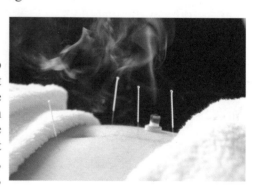

One of the main reasons that Tai Chi is so widely practiced in China is that it promotes a long and healthy life. The Taoists practiced a form of Tai Chi in their quest for eternal youth, and the doctor Sun Simiao, known throughout the Chinese world as the Medicine King, lived to the ripe old age of 100, conscientiously carrying out the forms. He recommended it as an excellent way of maintaining good health, urging his patients to learn perseverance and patience from the steady progress they made with Tai Chi.

Tai Chi is also a safe and practical sport. There is no risk of acute cardiac problems when practicing, and it is an excellent all-round healthy activity. Because of its balanced yet cyclical nature, there are no sudden movements or jolts to shock weak joints or muscles, the movement is gentle and constant, with no stops or starts. Breathing is kept slow and regular throughout the form, instead of forcing participants to gasp for breath or stop for a rest. It is extremely practical in that no special equipment or dedicated space is required - comfortable loose clothing is all you need, and a little time regularly. You can keep up Tai Chi even when you are away from home.

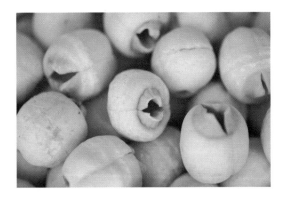

This activity can also improve general coordination, flexibility and mobility. This is especially true for older people. Regular Tai Chi sessions will strengthen the leg and back muscles reducing the likelihood of falls and injuries, giving more independence. Arthritis can be eased with regular practice, as Tai Chi can help strengthen the muscles around the affected joints, encouraging flexibility and enlarging the range of movements in a gentle, painless way. Tai Chi is suitable for all ages, irrespective of gender, physical condition or strength and ability. Like Yoga, those practicing Tai Chi go at their own pace without forcing any movements, each level providing room for improvement.

Tai Chi is fun and can be practiced alone or in a group, to soft music or in silence, indoors or out. The importance of enjoyable activity cannot be overstressed - relaxation and enjoyment are as important in life as work and study. The trick is to get the balance right - too much work makes Jack a dull boy! Even we in the west know that a healthy body means a healthy mind, and that happiness plays a major role in our health. And when it is practiced in a group, all the advantages of socialization and personal interaction are at play and the activity becomes something to look forward to. So tai chi can simply be practiced for fun, too, and to meet people.

Finally, Tai Chi can provide positive treatment for many serious illnesses.

According to the WHO, the main killers of our society are now cancer, heart diseases, brain diseases and diabetes. Tai Chi and TCM can be beneficial in the treatment of all of these.

In TCM cancer is believed to be caused by a deficiency of some kind, and tonic herbs such as Ginseng and Lingzhi (ganoderma mushroom) are usually prescribed. In Tai Chi, cancer is thought of as grains of sand in the muscles, and the gentle, smooth movements can help to ease them slowly out of the system.

The cardiovascular system can benefit greatly from the practice of Tai Chi, as this activity promotes overall circulation of blood. The leg muscles are worked extensively, thereby reducing the risk of blood clots or other problems affecting the extremities, and the overall benefit is that blood and oxygen are directed more regularly to the brain. In TCM, brain and heart problems are often treated with Dan Shen, in tea, powder or tablet form.

Diseases of the blood can be slowed down with certain teas: Jiang Zhi tea for reducing cholesterol, Jiang Tang tea for lowering blood sugar levels, and Jiang Ya for blood pressure. Regular Tai Chi sessions have been proven highly effective for improving the heart rate, especially for normally sedentary elderly people, and for reducing blood pressure by decreasing stress. The immune system can also be improved with Tai Chi.

As with TCM, Tai Chi works the body and mind as a whole, seeking to rebalance Yin and Yang. Where TCM treats with herbs, massage and acupuncture. Tai Chi works with movement. Both offer genuine health benefits.

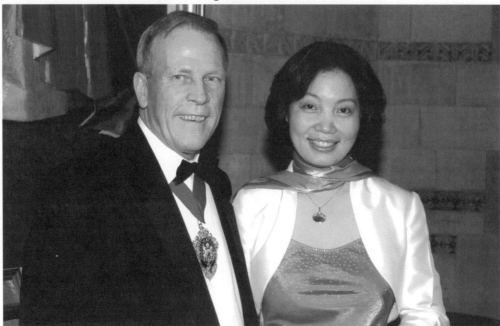

Prof. Shulan Tang with Lord Mayor of Manchester, Councillor Tom OCallagham in November 2004.

TAi CHi is A GREAT DISCIPLING FOR BOTH MIND AND BODY, AND A GOOD WAY TO KEEP FIT

CLLR Tom. OCallogh

Chapter Six:
Interviews With Practitioners
by Tim Birch

The following section includes a series of interviews with a cross section of Master Liming's students here in the U.K. The personal accounts provide descriptions of the experiences and personal benefits relating to the health aspect of practicing Chen Style Tai Chi. The students range from twenty-something's to octogenarians; from people who are just starting out in their first year to those with more than a decade of experience.

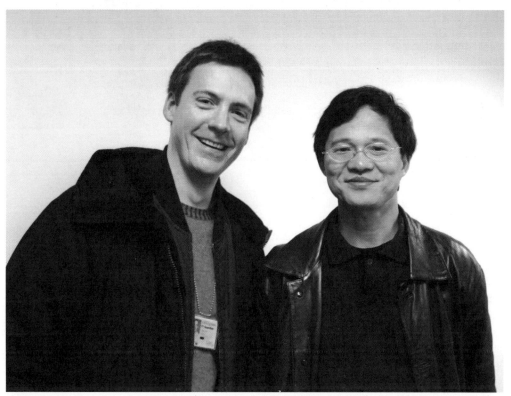

Master Liming Yue and Tim Birch meet up at the final interview for the book

The initial interviews were conducted with Master Liming Yue's senior students, some of whom have studied under Grandmaster Chen Zhenglei and are now teaching Chen Style Tai Chi in various parts of the British Isles. Additional interviews were conducted with individuals who are active in intermediate classes led by Master Liming Yue and Grandmaster Kongjie Gou, with the final selection of shorter interviews conducted with students from many of the foundation classes which are held by Master Liming Yue throughout the North West region. The interviewees were generous, candid and offer an invaluable insight into the multitude of benefits which are to be gained from regularly practicing Chen Style Tai Chi. Thanks are respectfully given to them.

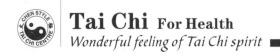

Dan Chisholm, 29; Full-time instructor of Chen Style Tai Chi based in West Sussex.

Q: When did you start Chen Style Tai Chi?

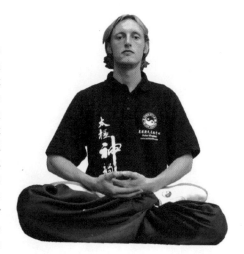

I began learning with Master Liming Yue in 1996 whilst studying at University in Manchester. I noticed an advertisement for new classes showing Master Liming Yue in an incredibly low posture and I knew from that moment I had to join. From the very first class there was no doubt that I had found someone special. Master Liming Yue has a control and gracefulness to his movements with an underlying presence of power that is jaw dropping. I have complete admiration for someone who has dedicated their life to achieve such a high level of skill and has inspired me to follow in his footsteps.

Q: So has it proved good fortune?

Definitely! I found out recently that my arrival in Manchester coincided with that of Master Liming's from China, so I guess I was just in the right place at the right time. You can call it fate, to meet such an accomplished teacher but it's important for the individual to recognize the opportunity and make full use of it.

I have been extremely fortunate to have only studied from some of the most talented masters in the world. Once you have witnessed and experienced this level of training anything else is just a disappointment. Life is short and Tai Chi is a long and challenging journey. To reach the highest levels it is essential that you find a good teacher who can guide and direct you along the correct path. If you are going to succeed in any activity it makes sense to learn from the most experienced practitioners available. This ensures you gain the maximum benefit and limits the amount of wasted time.

Q: What has kept you intrigued by Chen Style Tai Chi over time?

No matter what level you reach you will always find there is something more to learn. This is probably Tai Chi's greatest asset. Once you begin you will never become bored since all the benefits and abilities you develop become increasingly more profound as you progress. From relaxation to health, fitness to healing, martial application to spiritual training, all aspects are founded on the same basic principles that permeate every aspect of this art. It's just up to the individual how far you take it.

Tai Chi will continually challenge you physically and mentally. At first the movements seem easy to follow. But they require more than just simple replication. There is an underlying energy that needs to be stimulated, understood and then allowed to flow. But the whole process takes time. Once you learn to relax and listen to your body, your internal energy begins to flow. This creates a fluidity of movement that could not be produced through simply using body mechanics alone.

Q: How would you summerize Chen Style Tai Chi?

Chen Style Tai Chi is a dynamic system of movement that adheres precisely to the original Taoist principles of Yin and Yang. A student should be able to perform all movements with a clear understanding of these elements, since without it true balance is impossible. Movements should be smooth, graceful and effortless due to the involvement of internal energy. Once this internal energy has been stimulated and flows unobstructed; optimum health, self-awareness, healing abilities, martial skill and spiritual understanding all become accessible.

Q: Have you had any health troubles?

No. I have been fortunate with my health but this is mainly due to being heavily involved in sports from a young age. Personally, I see Tai Chi as an essential daily supplement, like a vitamin, that is important in sustaining a healthy body. Softer forms of moderated exercise like Tai Chi are far more beneficial to long term health than the modern "impact" forms of exercise that seem to provide only short-term benefits and do little to protect the long-term health of the individual. Softer exercises like Tai Chi is finally being recognized as providing the greatest benefits to physical and mental health that are sustainable well into old age.

Tai Chi has continued to keep me healthy and flexible, both physically and mentally. The benefits to my own health develop the more I study and I have begun to lay the foundations for good health for the rest of my life.

Q: What, for you, are the key health gains from studying Chen?

I personally feel that the most important gain from practicing Chen Style Tai Chi is the ability to relax. Relaxation is the most fundamental requirement and the root from which all other benefits will stem. After the body and mind are able to relax, subtle and gradual changes begin to occur within the body. The combinations of relaxation with the subtle twisting actions of the movements produce similar effects to massage. These massaging actions remove toxins, replenish the supply of nutrient rich blood, and promote optimum health and vitality.

Q: So a key point is that Chen Style Tai Chi helps you to get in touch with your body?

Yes. I think it surprises people just how much you start to understand your body and how your mind plays a role in effecting your state of health. These so-called "simple exercises" help to calm the mind, strengthen the body and allow you to develop a greater sensitivity and awareness of the self. Tai Chi is a deeply personal activity where everyone develops at a different rate as they begin to understand the feelings and sensations produced from practicing this fascinating art.

Q: Could you expand on the broader health benefits?

One of the most valuable features of practicing Tai Chi is its ability to calm the mind. The slow, meditative style of the movement provides the key for relieving tension and stress. Emotions, such as anger, anxiety and fear are the origin of many illnesses. Once emotions are brought under control by calming the mind, improvements to health begin to develop.

As the movements in Tai Chi are undertaken slowly, the body is gently conditioned to soften and tone all the muscles. This approach to training requires all the muscles to be exercised in a balanced and natural way that incorporates the whole body. This is essential to maintain good posture.

The movements performed during Tai Chi exercise lead to increased digestion, greater vitality, improved circulation, increased appetite, stabilized emotions and a calmer mind that will leave you feeling relaxed and refreshed - and all this from a simple exercise system!

Q: Any long-term reflections on Chen Style Tai Chi?

Tai Chi is not just a "simple exercise". It is a profound system that involves physical, mental and spiritual training. Little did I know when I attended my very first class that I would now be teaching and promoting this incredible art?

From my own training, I understand just how important Tai Chi can be in all aspects of life. It has allowed me greater control over my emotions and helped to develop a greater understanding of myself.

Unfortunately most people seem to take their health for granted, only becoming interested in healthcare after being confronted with illness. Keeping an active body and mind are essential to fight off ill health, senility and the multitude of problems that people associate with aging. With the right training, you can remain active and healthy well into your senior years, which is ironically, the part of your life when you have the time and the money to enjoy it.

Q: Any particular reflections on the mysterious internal aspect to Chen Style Tai Chi?

Tai Chi is a form of meditation that utilizes movement to develop spiritual awareness. Simple techniques are used to stimulate a feeling of internal energy. Once stimulated, the collection, circulation and refinement of this energy is required to strengthen the body and improve health. By practicing Tai Chi regularly energy begins to flow freely and movement becomes lighter and more fluid. By becoming sensitive to our bodies, energy is used to direct the flow of movement.

The closest analogy I can find to Tai Chi is mountain climbing. Most people aspire to reach the top. It ultimately comes down to talent, guidance and the individual's own determination to succeed. The journey can be long and challenging and some days we make great progress, whilst other days we will feel we are making no progress at all. There are thousands of steps and it is important that we should enjoy the views (benefits) along the way. Most importantly of all, we need to remind ourselves that the view from the summit is the best one. If we find times of difficulty or lose enthusiasm we must carry on. Each step, however insignificant, takes us one step closer to our final destination.

Ploutarchos Pluto Vlachopoulos, Chen Style instructor based in Athens, Greece.

Q: When did you start Chen Style Tai Chi?

I did kung fu for about a year and a half when I was 15 but it was not anything serious, it was mainly exercise. I was a track athlete. I did track for about four years 200m and long jump. So I always used to do exercise but Tai Chi was the first thing I have gone into seriously. I started Tai Chi in 2001. Master Liming Yue was my first teacher, it was weird because at some point I wanted to do something physical, a martial art. But of the martial arts I have known, I never really liked any of them. So I did a small search into Tai Chi. Also, I had met a lady who had advised me to do it if you find a good teacher. So, for me, meeting Master Liming Yue was fate.

Q: Is it key to find the right master?
Sure. And Master Liming Yue is the best in the UK and Europe.

Q: So you are highly committed to Chen Style Tai Chi?

Yes. I am doing Tai Chi as a discipline, as an art, from the health point-of-view and from the physical point-of-view. And one other reason now is the business point-of-view. I am putting much more emphasis on it. After the first year I went to China, I decided more or less not to do my MPhil but to go fully into Tai Chi. That I would do Tai Chi in Athens as a job. It is a small risk.

Q: What is your opinion of the health aspect to Chen Style Tai Chi?

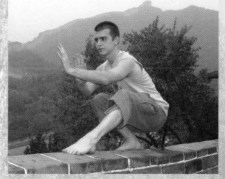

The one specific I can tell you is that during the time I have been doing Tai Chi I have become calmer. People who do not know me and people who do know me have told me, quite a few times, that I emanate calmness. And I was not like that four or five years ago. I was more nervous, tense. Tai Chi has definitely helped to relax me. Also in my way of thinking. So I personally can speak for relaxation. If you practise Tai Chi you are definitely going to relax.

Q: How would you summerize the broad benefits to Chen Style?

The thing is, when you start practicing Tai Chi, depending on the person, sooner rather than later you start to feel the Qi inside your body. It can improve your physical well-being without you noticing it: Things like agility, joints [suppleness], flexibility, balance and coordination of movements. Your body starts to become more aware of positioning such as the placing of the hands. And all of that simultaneously trains your mind because it is a mind exercise as well. Because once you start feeling something, you have to think about it. If you do not think about it then it has gone. You have to concentrate on what you are doing. So Tai Chi also helps concentration. There are many aspects to health. And generally, if you have a particular problem like a knee problem or waist problem or neck problem, you are not sleeping well, headaches, migraines, back problems, etc... all that, while practicing Tai Chi, problems are eased or made better.

Q: Has your experience of a more intensive training schedule led to acute developments?

Rapid. I mean, I started as everyone else doing Tai Chi once a week. But even with that, I saw some difference in the first few months. It depends on the person because someone might be more physical so he can take more exercise and so he will feel the effects of Tai Chi sooner rather than later. In the West, people often think about benefits and how soon can I have it. So when you start a gym it is about how fast you are going to lose weight, etc. Tai Chi is not like that. The short term benefit comes as soon as you start feeling the energy and so you start getting into the exercise. Then as time goes by, depending on your training and your effort, the longer term benefits can grow substantially and exponentially.

Q: What sets Chen Style Tai Chi apart in your estimation?

A lot of people do not realize that Tai Chi is actually Kung Fu. It is the original style of Kung Fu, I mean it is one of the earliest, basic forms of Kung Fu. Chen Style is the original style of Tai Chi. From Chen Style, all the other four branches of Tai Chi -Yang, Wu, Wu and Sun- have been developed. I have to admit I have not done any of the other styles, but I have seen Yang Style and spoken with people who did Yang Style and Chen Style. For me, the basic difference is that with Chen you can feel much more the martial art application. And you feel like you are doing martial arts together with, how can I put it, health exercise. Again depending on the person, you can put more emphasis either on the health or the martial arts aspect of Chen Style Tai Chi. Someone who puts more effort on the martial side gets the benefit of the health as well because it is the same exercise and vice versa. One of the main differences is that the energy releases are missing in the other styles. With Chen, and maybe it is because it is the original style, you can feel the energy, the Qi, sooner and stronger, perhaps. I think that is the case.

Q: Could you shed some light on the internal side to Chen Style?

Tai Chi internal side is like a separate category of the martial arts. You can learn Kung Fu, the moves, the kicks, the spins and all that in quite a short time if you really put effort into it. But the thing is, manipulating your energy, your Qi, is a whole different thing. You have to do it by practicing exercises. But it is also something you have to do by mind, so it is a lot different than the external martial arts only because of that internal aspect of Qi and how you can manipulate it and how can you make it either help your body or indeed others.

Martin Millar, 58, Office Manager based in Manchester.

Q: Could you outline your route into Chen Style Tai Chi?

I am in my second career at present. Previously I was a police officer in Manchester for 33 years. I have always kept fit. In my youth I played rugby and when I got too old for that I kept the physical side of my activities going. I worked out regularly for many years jogging and weight training. Although I was physically active I had a traumatic experience some years ago. I went to my doctor for a minor ailment and he gave me the news that I had suffered a heart attack. And that stopped me in my tracks. After various tests they decided that it was a very minor one. He was never happy about my weight training and he advised me against it. But he encouraged me to take up a physical activity, because, as part of my condition, I suffer from hypertension, or high blood pressure. So I had to get some physical activity. My son had recently started practicing Tai Chi. I knew nothing about it. Through him I found out it was good for 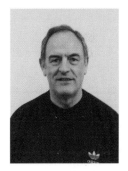 hypertension. Although my son did Tai Chi, my impression of it was old dears waving their hands about on the banks of the Yangtze. Though I had a condition I was not ready for that until I saw my son practicing on my back lawn. Then I realized the Tai Chi that he was practicing had nothing to do with old ladies waving their arms about in the air. So I read up on Tai Chi and decided that I would go with him to one of Liming's classes. That was 2002 and I have been coming ever since.

Q: So what were your initial impressions of Tai Chi?

I felt a benefit from the breathing. I felt better for it, I felt healthier. And it also helped me relax and certainly reduced my blood pressure. Now I practice a couple of times a week at home and I come to the classes regularly. I am really convinced that there is something in Tai Chi I have certainly benefitted from it.

Q: What, for you, is the everyday benefit from Tai Chi?

The everyday benefit of Tai Chi is that I am able to relax. I can practice Qigong breathing at work when I feel I am getting stressed. I can do these breathing exercises which I feel helps me to relax.

Q: What health benefits do you sense when practicing Chen Style?

When doing Tai Chi I feel I am exercising my heart, my lungs, and my body although not as physically as some of the exercises I have done. But I am no spring chicken anymore and I have to be aware that I can not get my body into some of the positions which I could when I was a younger man. But on the whole I feel the exercising in Tai Chi benefits me physically and, certainly, being able to relax benefits me mentally.

Q: So do you see Tai Chi as a kind of total health system?

I would not say it was the total health system but there is something there and I benefit from it personally so I continue to do it. I just feel I am benefitting from it and yet there is more to come.

Q: Better to call it a complimentary health system?

All I can say is there is something in it which I do not understand.

Alastair Macgillivray, aged 55, a working G.P. from Hyde.

Q: When did you start practicing Chen Style Tai Chi?

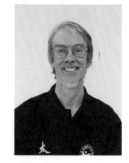

I have been practicing Yang style for about three or four years and I have been learning this style [Master Liming's Chen Style], which is more difficult, for about 8 months. It's quite vigorous really - but I enjoy it. And it's fantastic value. Liming is a fantastic teacher.

Q: How do you fit Tai Chi into the busy schedule of a G.P.'s life?

The pressures of work are there but to make a change you've got to really want to do it. Tai Chi is part of my normal working day now and so I try to reorganise my schedule around this class.

Q: Given your professional life as a G.P., why do you practice Tai Chi?

I think medicine does not answer all the questions. And it is nice to be able to do something of your own effort towards getting better or to being better.

Q: Do you recommend Tai Chi in your work as a G.P.?

Yes. A lot of people come to see me, virtually every surgery, complaining of stress. So, in terms of Tai Chi, let`s take `breathing` as our example. We can focus on our breathing by just breathing deeper while making slight movements. If you breathe with a slight hand movement it gives you a timing; a pace. It helps people focus. I`ve always been encouraging people to breathe more deeply to relax, ever since I was in practice, for over twenty years. If you breathe more deeply you get more energized.

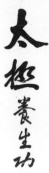

Q: You mentioned 'stress' and, these days, we're constantly being told from various sources that stress is sharply increasing with our 'ever faster lifestyles'. Could Tai Chi be a tonic for stress?

You used to be able to refer 'people with significant anxiety' for relaxation therapies, but the Mental Health Service, now, will hardly accept any referrals. So, there are some local Tai Chi classes, in Hyde and my patients have had good results since they started Tai Chi. They're actually helping others by running classes for other patients.

Q: In your considered opinion, how does Tai Chi benefit people?

It's really for the people to get out of it what they want. It's trying to oversimplify it to put it into particular benefits. In life you experience certain things and if the experience makes you feel better, and you can reproduce that feeling, then 'the thing' is good. With Tai Chi, you really get out of it what you put into it. I mean, you can read a book and it's nice but if you keep reading it, it's perhaps not quite as intense whereas with Tai Chi it gets better. There are not many things that you can say that about.

Q: How would you summerize Tai Chi?

I think, ultimately, Tai Chi is an experience. So I would encourage anyone reading this to go and experience Tai Chi. It's something that you get more out of if you go and experience it. You need to go four or five times. Once you've done that, you've got over the initial 'what is this all about?' and begin to feel attuned to it.

Geoff Leversedge, 45; College Manager and part–time Chen Style instructor based in Norwich.

Q: When did you start Chen Style Tai Chi?

I have been doing Tai Chi, and supposedly Chen Style, for about twelve years. But I have now been with Liming for the last four years. And I have got to say, that was when my proper Tai Chi learning started. Basically I had been wandering in the wilderness for a while looking for a good teacher, then Liming came along.

Q: Why has learning with Master Liming proved significant?

It is the same with everything there are going to be better and poorer quality in terms of the teaching that is going. Now I have always believed that the closer you are to the source of the family side of things then the better chance you have of actually getting the authentic teaching. Master Liming has been trained by Grandmaster Chen Zhenglei and others, so what we get from Liming is very close to the source. And that is important because things do get diluted as with all the martial arts.

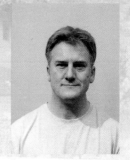

Q: What has been your general experience of the health aspect to Chen Style?

Very positive. Before I started Chen Style I was very fit. I played squash and football. I thought Tai Chi was going to be a doddle. But it was actually one of the hardest things I ever started to learn. Because I realized, very early on, that I was not flexible. That I was not as fit as I thought I was.

Q: Do you have a specific insight into the health benefits?

I had a football injury before I took up Tai Chi. It was my lower spine right on the coccyx. I could still play football but as soon as I started to bend in the waist I seized up, I could barely get my hands to about knee height. With regular stretching and everything else with Tai Chi, palms are now flat on the floor. You see, half the time you do not realise that you are carrying injuries or aches and pains. I had been getting these football injuries which did not seem to be good things to take into my old age. I took up Tai Chi not knowing what it could do and found that even though I did not seem to be working as hard, I was getting a lot more benefit from the type of exercise.

Q: So what do you see as distinguishing Tai Chi exercise?

I see the difference between West and East. There is an awful lot of compression of muscles and joints in Western training like weight lifting and not so much of the stretching aspects which really do come out in things like Tai Chi and yoga. The stretching seems, from a physical point of view, to have an enormous benefit in terms of getting rid of the aches and pains and everyday things like bad posture or not being able to touch your toes which sound silly but the knock-on effects are quite profound.

Q: What kind of knock-on effects have you noticed from practicing Chen Style?

Energy wise, enormous increases. As time went on and the practice became better then a good session of Tai Chi would see me, say, clubbing into the early hours of the morning when my colleagues had given up a few hours before I mean, those are the silly anecdotal things which come to mind.

Given that you also teach Chen Style, how would you summerize it?

An awful lot of people believe that Tai Chi is all gentle: the soft gentle movements in the park stuff. So the shock to the system for a lot of people is that is only one aspect to the training. There is a huge amount to the training. Through Tai Chi, you will become much more analytical about your own body. I mean we do not pay much attention in the West to what we do with our bodies, we tend to be really bad at putting our bodies into uncomfortable positions and so on. With Tai Chi you will learn about how your body works and its functionality and will therefore be able to do things to help it.

Q: What are the everyday benefits of practicing Chen Style?

Through working with the body in Tai Chi, you get to know your own body very, very well. Because you are inwardly analyzing what you are doing you tend to be able to pinpoint, after a while, exactly where a particular problem might be focused. And as a result of using your Tai Chi training and exercise, daily, you can work on that particular area to actually improve it.

Q: What of the longer term benefits with Chen Style?

A lot of people come to my classes because they have heard that it is good for health but do not really have a clue what is involved. It is the same with anything that you do: you need to put in the practice in order to get the benefits. And nobody should be under the illusion that it is going to be a quick fix. It is not like these adverts that say something like tummy trimmed in two months or whatever. Benefits you will get, but only if you put the effort in. And the benefits with Tai Chi seem to last longer because it is stretching. If you stretch a tendon it tends to stay stretched longer than a muscle which, once it has been worked and then relaxed, tends to turn to fat quicker."

Q: Do the health benefits of Tai Chi apply to all ages?

They do apply to people of all ages. I firmly believe that... I have one class of old ladies in sheltered housing. The oldest one there is 92. I have only been with them about six months but, now, all of the ladies come into the room with a spring in their step. They are very chatty, lively, very keen on it. Their practice is obviously limited given their ages and bodies, but they are getting something out of it even at their age. Whilst the Tai Chi is tempered for what their bodies can actually take, they are experiencing benefits out of it. In terms of their dedication, their interest, and how I can see the benefits are hitting them, I have to say that they are a remarkable group. It is proved to me that it does not matter what age you come to this. Even if their mobility is not hugely improved, their minds are more active. It really has given them a new lease of life, if you like.

Q: In your overall estimation, what is special about Chen Style?

I have got to say that Chen Style Tai Chi is one of the most mentally demanding things I have ever undertaken. It is intellectually challenging because of your battle with your body. You make your body do things that it is not used to doing. And there is quite a big mental challenge to this. So from a holistic point of view, it is that never-ending mental challenge along with the physical challenge which gives the complete picture, and makes it special.

Anthony Rushton, aged 35. Martial arts instructor based in Malvern, Worcester.

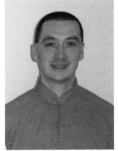

Q: When did you start training in the martial arts?

I first started training in the martial arts and fitness at around the age of 9. Learning what I could from friends, books, films and anything else I could find to help me. But my first Martial arts class was in the art of Wing Chun

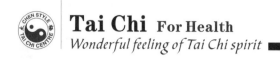

Kung Fu. An excellent style. I have also studied other great arts along the way. I love all arts and the way they work so well together.

Q: When did you start Chen Style Tai Chi?

About five years ago I saw an advert of Master Liming Yue's. I spoke with him and bought some of his videos. I learned intensively, as much as I could, from the tapes and then visited him and had a lesson. I was hooked. I have continued to see him five or six times a year. It varies but I consider him my master."

Q: How has Tai Chi benefitted you in terms of health?

The stance work has helped my lower back problems. Helping me to relax. As at that time I was in a lot of pain. Master Liming Yue, also gave me some exercises to do, additionally. This helped a great deal.

Q: Any related health benefits?

Yes. My lower back and inner groin feel much better. I now have a new allover feeling of goodness.

Q: So Chen Style Tai Chi is proving a good complementary system for you?

Chen Style is an excellent complementary system for me and works so well with my training in other styles.

Steven Burton, aged 33, Professional Martial Arts Instructor based in Accrington Lancashire.

Q: Background?

I started martial arts when I was eight years old and I settled with Shaolin Kung Fu, the Southern Kung Fu style Lau Gar. I'm currently a guardian of that style making sure that standards are maintained. I have been studying that for 20 years. I also hold a black belt grade in kick boxing and an Okinawan art called Torite Jutsu.

Q: Tai Chi?

I'd had some exposure of Yang Style Tai Chi through my Lau Gar Kung Fu master. And once I'd studied the Yang Style I wanted to find a tai chi master and I came across Liming. I started Chen Style around 1998 studying with Liming. I started with one of his intensive courses then started classes and branched into having private lessons with Liming. More recently I've also studied with Grandmaster Gou and I've gone over to China, studying with Grandmaster Chen Zhenglei.

Q: So given that you're a professional martial arts instructor, what attracted you to Chen Style?

Tai Chi attracted me for the philosophical side and the health aspect. I was fortunate in coming across Liming as once I'd trained with him, and having experience of training with other highly skilled Chinese Masters in other Chinese arts, I was aware that he really knew what he was talking about and his level of skill was just fantastic. Liming had some background in Shaolin Kung Fu so we were both talking the same language as it were. I just really liked Liming's approach to teaching, the way he portrayed the knowledge and his attention to detail.

I was also aware of the health aspects to Tai Chi, so more recently I've studied specific aspects of Qigong with Liming as well. He just seemed to have the whole package: the quality of teaching and the level of knowledge and understanding of the art, also having the direct recognition, the credibility of the lineage in which he's trained. Liming has a very credible lineage because his teachers have been Grandmaster Chen Zhenglei and Grandmaster Kongjie Gou.

Q: have you joyed good health?

My good level of health has been relatively consistent. Through my gaining of Chinese concepts through Liming, and my other teachers, I actually lecture on Chinese medical concepts regarding to Tai Chi at the University of Central Lancashire, the honours degree course in Complimentary Medicine. But my understanding has been developed a lot more since training with Liming.

Q: So as an instructor of Chen Style, what are the health benefits you've observed in others?

I have some 200 plus students in Tai Chi around East Lancashire, varying in age from teenagers. Recently we had a lady who was 107. I do modified versions in a seated form. And I work quite closely with the Health and Fitness Development Department of Blackburn Borough Council improving balance, flexibility, coordination and mobility. People find that through practicing it also helps boost the immune system -through some of the Qigong breathing exercises. It's a general sense of well being. People who suffer depression and various things like that tend to find that it gives them lift. Some of the exercises, on the medical implication side of things, cause the body to produce certain hormones such as seratonin and dopamines, the things which basically make you happy. Certain Qigong exercises can cause that 'happy' effect in people so I find that people who suffer depression have had great benefit from practicing the exercises. I could go on and on with the number of people I've trained. People who suffer arthritis have had

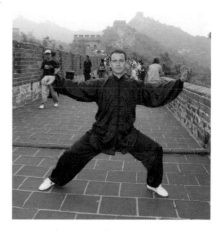

tremendous gain. Particularly, in my experience, people with osteoarthritis seem to gain quicker results. Although everybody with arthritis can gain some results people with rheumatoid arthritis gain benefits but it just takes a little bit longer.

Q: How do you advise on the practice of Chen Style in our busy world?

I would definitely say to practice as little and often as is available. Even if it is five or 10 minutes a day, it'll certainly contribute towards people's health. I mean I like to look at medical principles and that perspective but, generally, a sense of well being is what people find from practicing. The sense of feeling calm and collected. Certainly the Qigong and Tai Chi tends to give you that calming type of feeling so that you learn to step back in a difficult situation, take a few breaths, and then look at it objectively. Like clearing your head before you go and solve problems. Personally, I'm so hectic with the school that I have and I dash round the country teaching, I tend to find that it keeps my head clear and it keeps me form getting stressed. One of the phrases I always use is that 'Tai Chi is keeping your body young as you get older.'

Q: Could you expand on that?

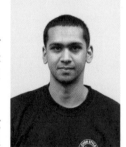

It just keeps you young. It keeps everything mobile. For me, I genuinely want to live in excess of 100, but I want my health to go with it and I personally believe that Tai Chi will do that.

Aamir Rafi, 22, Chen Style Instructor, completing BSc (Hons) Exercise & Health Sciences at Salford University, based in Manchester

Q: Did you have a background in martial arts before taking up Chen Style?

I started in 1998 with traditional Shaolin Kung Fu and I dabbled a bit in Chang Chuan. I've done bits of Western boxing and mixed martial arts. But basically I've got a lot of my foundation from the Shaolin Kung Fu.

Q: How did you make the transition to Chen Style Tai Chi?

Well one of my Shaolin teachers had practiced Chen Style with Chen Zhenglei. But he was more on the external side of things. So I found Liming and went to one of his classes in 2001. And I've stuck with him ever since.

Q: How do you find training with Master Liming?

He's opened up a lot of stuff, especially relating to the Shaolin forms as well as the martial applications. So it's not just the Chen Style.

Q: How do you personally define Chen Style?

I see it as a martial art. I understand it's been portrayed as a health exercise because it has many health benefits. For example, correct practice of it doesn't stress the body. Actually it heals the body, by correcting the alignment of the bones and improving your breathing. But, overall, I see it as an art form, a martial art form.

Q: Have you always had good health?

Generally, yeah. I've had my medial cartilage removed from my left knee. That was caused by a lot of jumping, landing, twisting and kicking. I don't feel it at all since I've done Tai Chi. Actually I sort of used the Tai Chi as rehabilitation to get me back to my strenuous Shaolin training but I've stayed with the Tai Chi. And my leg's a lot better, a lot stronger.

Q: What everyday health benefits have you experienced with Chen Style?

I'm more aware of my body. It sounds strange because I've always been quite active and aware. But, still, I'm more aware of bad things like slouching and good things like 'sinking down'. I'm just more sensitive about parts of my body, like relaxing my shoulders. A common cause of stress is tense shoulders causing headaches. I feel more energetic generally, just more fresh every day. If I lack sleep certain nights, I still feel quite energetic the next day.

Q: And can you pinpoint any longer term benefits?

The Qigong breathing massages your internal organs so it increases their function. So as you practice more, and as you grow older, your health stays more balanced rather than fluctuating.

Q: So how would you personally sum up Chen Style?

Basically, Tai Chi is a philosophy which is based on certain principles. So it doesn't really matter about the certain moves that you do. As long as the principles are correct, so that they can be applicable to martial arts and health.

Grandmaster Kongjie Gou, aged 60; Full-time Instructor of Chen Style Tai Chi based in Manchester, UK

Q: Could you start by recounting, in brief, your personal story and experience of Tai Chi?

Tai Chi to me is the unforgettable exercise of my life. I would never give it up. I did try other Martial Arts in the past but I found that Tai Chi has the most effective benefits for me -particularly when I had cancer when I was young. I had a strong belief I could use Tai Chi to fight the cancer and stay alive, keeping a good health for the future. I very strongly believed this. It comes from the Tai Chi philosophy which is to believe sincerely and strive for higher motivation, otherwise you won't have any chance to win against something like cancer. I convinced myself that I had such good Tai Chi that I would not die. I believed that I wouldn't die. I just kept practicing. This is why I've practiced for 35 years. I have had very good health and a very good mental state -a happy mood. A further benefit is that although my body is small compared to the average person, I have been able to use intelligent application of Tai Chi skill. And though I have been challenged by many other Martial Artists in the past I have never been beaten. This is the Martial Arts benefit of the Tai Chi skill.

Q: And now, how are you personally gaining from Chen Style Tai Chi?

I have a very healthy mental state. This is a crucial point, the psychological side. When you practice Tai Chi you should pay more attention to the mental and spiritual side, not the muscular side. You use the mental to control the physical, that is your body's movements. I have a very settled mental state. I use mind control.

Q: What, other than mind control, is key to someone beginning to understand Chen Style Tai Chi?

The circular movements in Tai Chi. The spiral shapes. These help you to relax the body so you have no blockages. So everything is flowing smoothly: Blood, breath, energy and Qi. This is key. You will have better health. And everything is based on good health.

Q: How do you explain Tai Chi and its health benefits?

Tai Chi is one kind of Martial Arts exercise. It has great Martial Arts applications and benefits. But all the Martial Arts application is based around having good health and body condition. This is fundamental to Tai Chi. All the skill is based on good health. For example, how can you fly to China if you don't have the ticket? How can you practice so hard and not have benefits to everything, breathing, muscles, relaxation. Those kinds of benefits come from harder training. But if it's harder, it's also harder to catch cold, and other sicknesses because your body is stronger.

Q: Could you explain further about the movements and exercises?

Tai Chi movements are soft and flowing, and the benefits from this are that it makes your body very flexible and relaxed, with more sensitivity. This describes the top half of the body. The lower half of the body is very settled and solid. It looks like a tree with the tops blowing in the wind and the trunks rooted.

Q: So does the tree metaphor summerize the actual benefits as well as 'the look' of Tai Chi?

Yes in terms of development. Tai Chi perfectly suits the natural human growth of getting old, older and weaker, because Tai Chi offers the opposite benefits as you age. You get fitter and younger. The reverse of getting old. Whereas the natural procedure of aging is getting stiff, Tai Chi keeps you flexible. My conclusion is that Tai Chi 'fights age back'.

Q: What about the ostensibly 'invisible', internal benefits?

Another benefit is a change in the way of breathing. Normal breathing uses the lung and Tai Chi breathing goes lower, to the Dantian. As deeper, longer breathing equals more oxygen supply and increased lung capacity. More efficiency. This ties in with all of Tai Chi's open-and-close movements. Plus the breathing, coupled with the movements, actually massages all your internal organs.

Q: What are your conclusions, at this stage of your life, regarding Chen Style Tai Chi?

First, Tai Chi can change your motivation - your mental state. You always look forward. I never become very depressed. Second are the body functions. Joints, muscles, everything is improved. Third is the breathing system, breathing is improved. These are the key benefits gained from Tai Chi that lead to a very good health and mental state with no external physical sickness at all. Such that, overall, people are getting fitter, gaining increased resistance and living longer, healthier lives.

Q: What's your general view of Tai Chi practice among people in the UK and beyond?

I notice a lot of people love Martial Arts and practice Tai Chi but it still has not been brought out, and explained, widely enough. Still a lot of people do not recognize the benefits of Tai Chi: its health and self-defence benefits. In particular, most people don't understand the deep meaning of Tai Chi and the real benefit you can get from it. People misconstrue the surface representation of Tai Chi, the waving of arms. This is just the basic understanding of it. There's more beneath the surface, great benefits. Tai Chi is a great exercise. No other sports exercise can replace it. It's so unique as the whole body works together: internal, external, extremities and roots, surface and deeper, and so on. All is together in one unit, even your hair with your internal organs. When one part of your body moves, all other parts move together simultaneously. When one part stays still, the others are still. All the movements are in harmony. But if many people here don't realize or know what Tai Chi is, then this just leads us to do more promotion to let everybody understand the Tai Chi philosophy to a higher level. My wish is for most people to recognize the great benefits of Tai Chi for health, self-defence and fitness. Tai Chi is growing healthily and it will prove beneficial to more and more people in the future. I treat the Tai Chi as seeds, hopefully growing up with flowers and good results in the future.

太極養生功

Q: Now that you are based in Manchester, UK, how do you foresee your work here?

My emphasis will be on training the younger generation from a young age in a very good system. Serious training starts from very young. Everybody will become very professionally, skillful. So one aim is to build a group of young people so that those people can spread the benefits of Tai Chi and influence others. That's a key focus. Also I aim to train a group talented and interested students to become instructors. I wish to help more people become qualified to teach Chen Style Tai Chi, again to help promote Tai Chi. I also hope to create a core group of Tai Chi practitioners in the Chen Style Tai Chi Centre who will go around and do demonstrations and performances as part of the promotion of Tai Chi. To let people see Tai Chi in a straightforward way and to spread its teachings.

Plus, of course, this work opportunity benefits me as I get older. Having moved from China to Manchester, UK, I have come to a good environment. I can work as a full-time instructor in the Chen Style Tai Chi Centre and this is very good for my retirement.

What of the future?

I'm doing a job I'm interested in. And as I can train so much, I can expect myself to improve my own Tai Chi to even higher standards!

BRIEF INTERVIEWS WITH PRACTITIONERS

The following interviews were conducted during an afternoon session of Tai Chi at the Age Concern Centre, Ashton, Tameside with Master Liming Yue.

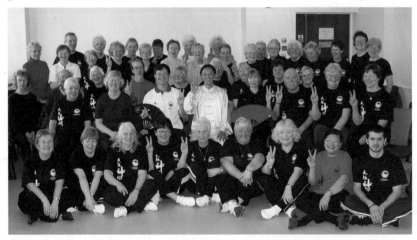

A group photo taken during the demonstration by Grandmaster Kongjie Gou and Master Liming Yue whilst the interviews took place with a group of students from AGE Concern in 2004

Dora Garlick, aged 74, retired actress.

When did you start Chen Style Tai Chi?

In 2003. Sixteen years ago I lost my husband with cancer and I had to get out so I joined a Tai Chi class and an art class. It was a different form of Tai Chi. I did it about three years and then they closed the school down unfortunately. It's over 10 years since I've done any Tai Chi. So I had to start over when I came to Age Concern, to the Tai Chi class here.

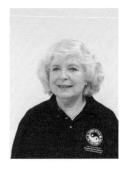

How does Tai Chi benefit you?

I feel much better since I joined it. My bones don't crack the same. When I come out of this class I feel buoyant and, you know, really well. It's good for your mind and bones and everything. We're all old but I find everyone has a similar experience of Tai Chi's benefits.

Ms Peebles, Age 65, Voluntary Worker for Age Concern.

When did you start Chen Style Tai Chi?

I came to do the classes first of all and then I got roped into being a volunteer. This is my third session, we do 12 week sessions.

How does Tai Chi benefit you?

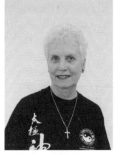

I'm a lot better since we started doing it. I have arthritis of the spine so it's helped me such a lot. I hardly have any pain with it now. My pain was very bad in the lower part of the back but since I've been doing this I've hardly suffered with it at all. It also shows you how to relax so it benefits you in a lot of ways. And I enjoy it!

Mary Johnson, retired Local Government Officer.

When did you start Chen Style Tai Chi?

I started four years ago but the class was discontinued. So I came to Liming's class last September [2003].

How does Tai Chi benefit you?

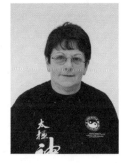

Well I've got very bad arthritic knees and feet and it helps with that because the exercise that we do helps the fluid that runs down the side of your knee and that helps. They don't hurt as much. Some of the other benefits I feel are in the things Liming teaches. He taught us a specific exercise with your ears which is good for inner balance. It sounds silly but this [tapping behind the ears] affects your spinal column - it reverberates right down your back. Now I used that on a plane and my ears didn't hurt. Also I like the calming influence that Tai Chi brings. I like the fluid movement. I've certainly got a lot more flexible since I did it. My feet and my knees don`t hurt anything like as much.

Irene Beech, retired Personal Assistant, UMIST.

When did you start Chen Style Tai Chi?

I used to go to a gym when I was working and I did a little bit of it. And now I'm retired I want to keep fit. I've only just joined.

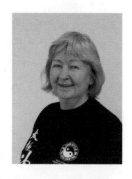

How does Tai Chi benefit you?

I was surprised at its gentleness at first, yet these movements were using muscles. My legs ached a bit. But I'm really getting into the flowing movements and enjoying them. I feel that my co-ordination, even though I've only been doing this a little while, has improved. I mean, when I first started I couldn't do a thing like Liming did, but now I find that the movements are becoming natural. I want to get more into that flow.

Sylvia Dearden, Age 64, retired Word Processor Operator.

When did you start Chen Style Tai Chi?

I went to another class for about two and a half years before coming to Liming. I've been here six months or something like that.

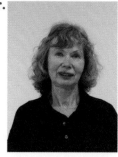

How does Tai Chi benefit you?

It helps me because I've got rheumatoid arthritis and I'm very stiff in the morning and I get quite a lot of pain at different times. But the movement of Tai Chi helps you, gently, to work all through your body, your muscles and tendons and everything. It just helps you to move better. Mobility is a key thing, for me, and Tai Chi has really helped. Plus, I go for blood tests every six months and when I was measured last he [the health practitioner] said, 'you've grown.' I said, 'I haven't', you shrink when you're getting older. But he was right. I'm 64 now but I'm standing better, my posture is better, I look like I've grown a bit. But it's the alignment of my spine. With standing better and getting everything in its right place I've grown a bit! All through doing Tai Chi. Alignment of your body is very important in Tai Chi. You do it unconsciously after you've been doing Tai Chi a while and you don't realize, perhaps, what bad posture you had before. I mean, in my thirties I couldn't walk about very well because of my knees being so painful. But I'm better in my sixties, quite honestly, for mobility, through Tai Chi I think. There are benefits that you don't realize until you think back, perhaps, before you started doing it. Balance, for example. I can go and try a shoe on now and balance on one leg. So my balance has improved tremendously because, with my knees, I'd have had to have sat down to try a shoe on before Tai Chi.

Iain Campbell, aged 68.

When did you start Chen Style Tai Chi?

I was starting to have problems with arterial blockage, and problems with balance, like staggering. In general, bad health, you know. So I started Tai Chi just over two years ago, incredible difference.

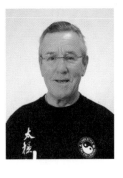

How does Tai Chi benefit you?

Well I'd had a heart attack in 1997 and became diabetic. But what an amazing recovery I've made since starting Tai Chi, you know. I've been back for several heart scans and the improvement has been tremendous. I've not said anything to them about Tai Chi but I know where the benefits are coming from, what with the meditation as well. My health has improved enormously.

Gwyn Fleetwood, aged 71, Professional Singer and Actor.

When did you start Chen Style Tai Chi?

About twelve months ago. I have done a lot of keep-fit and weight training in the past but I have never done Tai Chi.

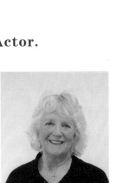

How does Tai Chi benefit you?

The benefits are that I have lost 2 stone and I just love it. I feel much healthier. My bones are much better. I can walk further. You see I joined Age Concern to go and see my brother, who is 84 to sit with him and have a cup of tea, you know. So then he told me about the Tai Chi and so I joined and it went on from there. I mean it is not only the things Liming teaches you. How can I say it? You just feel better relaxed, a life is worth living sort of feeling. You just feel good. And I feel great!

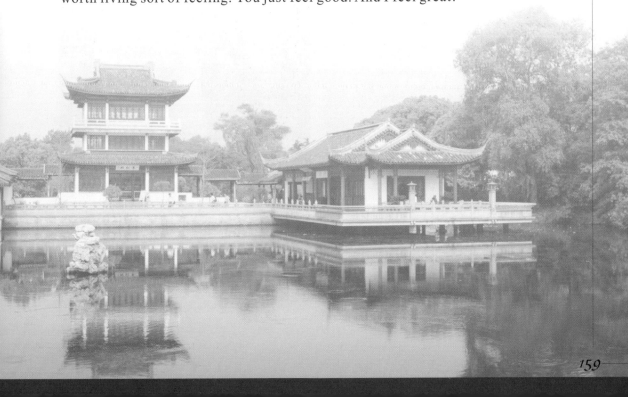

Chapter Seven
Dialogues with Master Liming Yue
All the answers to the questions you want to ask
by Master Liming Yue with Danny Chisholm
Nick Taylor and Anthony Rushton

Q1: *You have a very close professional relationship with Grandmaster Chen Zhenglei. What are the main ingredients required to strengthen the bond / relationship between student and teacher?*

A: The main ingredients that will form the basis of a good relationship with not only your teacher, but with any other people are: honesty, trust and respect. With your teacher you also require learning skills, capability, dedication and motivation. One of the main reasons that Grandmaster Chen Zhenglei and I have such a strong bond is because we think very much along the same lines. We do everything that we can, with wholehearted dedication, to promote the art of Chen Style Taijiquan to let people across the world receive the unique benefits of the authentic Chen Style Taijiquan.

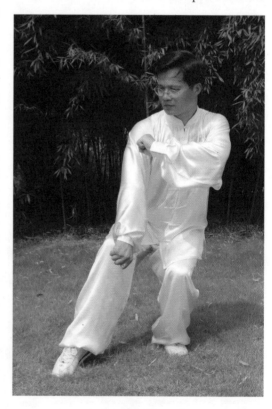

Q2: *Is the training in the Chen family village very different from any other parts of the world that practice Chen Style Taijiquan?*

A: There is quite a big difference. In the Chen Tai Chi village the training is very strict and a lot of emphasis is placed on the Martial Arts fighting application of the movements. This is combined with the great internal Qigong sensation feeling within the body for both health and self-defense. The instructors will come straight over to you and correct you on the spot.

In the village, everything has to be exactly right, being repeated over and over again until the master is happy.

Then, and only then, you are allowed to go on and learn the next movement. This is what impressed me the most, the level of intensity. Outside of the Chen village this is only shown when a person has been training for quite some time, wishing to obtain a higher level. Before you are taught at this intensity, the teacher will correct your movements and postures very gently and softly.

Q3: *Please could you explain the best way to train Fajing (energy release) and why Chen Taijiquan places so much emphasis on it.*

A: When training for Fajing (energy release), the movements must always be done in a relaxed way with an instant tensing at the end, followed by an instant relaxation. This is all done within a split second. Starting off with long strikes and working down to just one inch away to releasing energy.

Fajing (energy release) requires all the power to come from the ground in a spiral twisting motion. Travailing up through the legs to the waist, then out to the extremities. Being released in a rolling in and rolling out motion with elastic shaking strength.

There are many ways to practice Fajing (energy release) in Chen Style Tai Chi and the following training methods are just some samples.

If you train empty handed Fajing (energy release) then practice striking a piece of cloth hanging up, using long and short strikes on the cloth. This will help to speed up and sharpen your Fajing striking ability. You can see and feel exactly what is going on as the energy of your strikes penetrate the cloth.

If you train with weapons then the three meter long pole is the best for Fajing (energy release). Using the same method of release as the empty hand by feeling the wave of power from the root to the very end of the pole.

Because Fajing (energy release) belongs to Yang aspect of Tai Chi, which is the opposite of Yin, it is very important to show both and understand them equally and know how to blend them at the right time.

Fajing (energy release) is very important for self-defense, as it is very powerful and direct. This is why Chen Style places so much emphasis on Fajing (energy release). On a lot of occasions an attacker can be stopped with only one Fajing strike movement. The shoulder and elbows are the most effective strikes that can be used on an attacker, as this is especially devastating when striking the chest area.

Apart from the Martial Arts benefits of Fajing (energy release), the Fajing (energy release) exercises will also help you to remove the blockages inside of your body along the acupuncture channels, free your inner energy with blood circulation and make your breathing system more efficient. It is also a good way to keep fit and maintain your body in good shape. That is why the Chen Style Tai Chi puts so much emphasis on the Fajing (energy release).

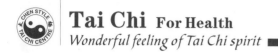
Q4: *Chen Style Taijiquan has a very good selection of weapons to train in. Which of these is your favorite and why?*

A: That will depend on what purpose you are intending to train for. For Fajing (energy release) I prefer the three-meter long flexible white wax pole.

For graceful, flexible and sensitivity Fajing (energy release) movements, I prefer sword and spear. The sword is called the king of the short weapons. It incorporates fast and slow continuous movements and can change direction very quickly as it is an extension of your arm and looks very beautiful in demonstrations. It is also an excellent defense weapon when you are situated in a limited space. The spear also requires the whole body to co-operate together but it needs much more space to practice.

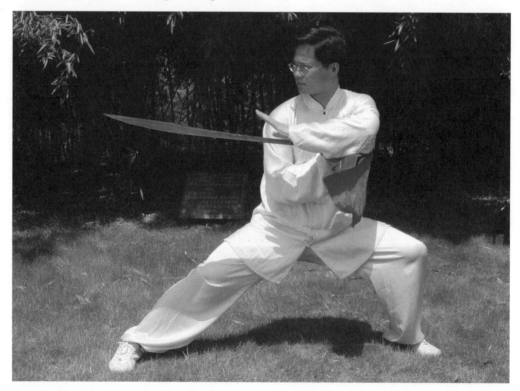

Q5: *What is Tai Chi Push Hands*

A: Push Hands is a practice method of traditional Tai Chi martial arts and a bridge connecting the movements with their applications. Two people with their arms in contact practice twining and sticking actions to develop the sense of touch, awareness and balance within the body. This is the training method where Tai Chi movements connect with martial arts applications and develops the understanding of how small forces can defeat strong physical power. There are five types of Push Hands method, which are Single Hand, Double Hand with fixed step, One Step forward and backward, Dalu (large step with low position) and Free-style Push Hands. It contains Peng, Lu, Ji, An and Cai, Lie, Zhou, Kao eight major Energy releasing methods, known in the West as Ward Off, Roll Back, Squeeze, Press and Pull Down, Cross Strike, Elbow, Shoulder.

Q6: *What should a person aim to achieve when first starting out in Taijiquan practicing Push Hands?*

A: For people who are interested in learning Push Hands, the first step is starting from Single Hand circling exercises then move onto the Double Hands Push Hands. The Double Hands Push Hands uses touching, turning and circling movements in the exercises, which will lead you to the stage of completion of the five main methods of Push Hands in the system.

At this level you should start to know the components of Push Hands while keeping in mind the mechanics of your own body. You learn the 'sticky' skills with the 'follow up' ability by rooting your own strength into the ground. Always make sure to balance yourself in a firm, strong and rooted stance for different positions or situations. You stay in touch with your opponent's arm by sticking whilst moving during the Push Hands exercise. This should increase your sensitivity to discover an opponent's strengths and weaknesses, creating attack or defense opportunities.

Q7: *What are the important issues for advanced level of practice Push Hands and applications?*

A: Use the mind to manage the body and movements without stiffness and any over-use of strength. The strength has to be no more than enough and no less than needed, just enough to support your movement and application. At this stage the following tips are highly recommended to Tai Chi practitioners:

Bend and Straight movements: Every time when you bend a limb (arm or leg) you immediately straighten it out again. The bend movements normally coincides with collecting and gathering energy, along with breathing in. Once the energy has been increased to the limit then this is the time to release it. You can do this quickly and with power by extending your arms out in a strike movement. Alternatively, extending your arm out in a strike but this time slowly, with mind, intent and consciousness playing a much bigger part. This will give the appearance of a slow gentle exercise charactistic of Tai Chi. N.B. Arms are never fully straightened.

Open and Close movements: In Tai Chi the Open movements mean stretching out your body or limbs and Close movements the opposite. Open is the beginning of the Close and Close is the beginning of the Open. When you open it will be followed by closing, and when you close it will be followed by

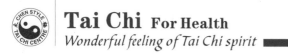
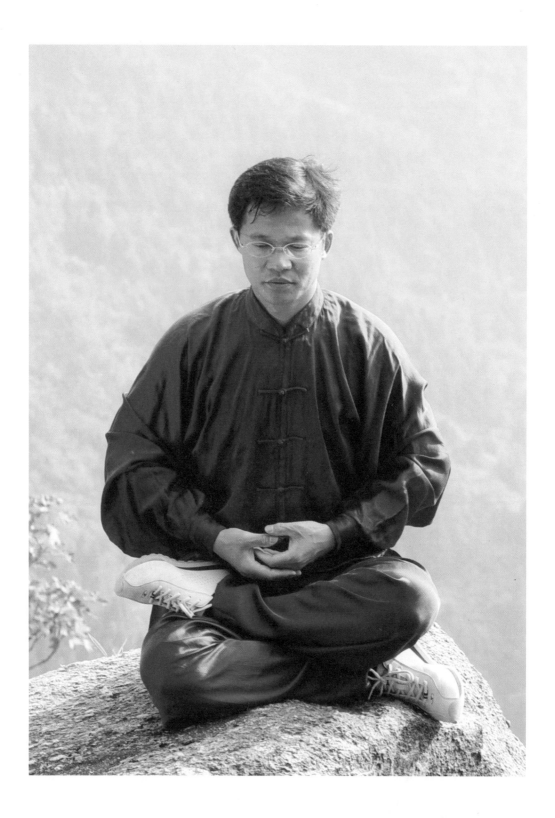

opening. Both open and close change into each other. Always push out or release energy whilst you are just closing.

Sticky and following up movements: Sticky means using your limbs (such as arms or legs) to stay in contact with your opponent all the time whilst you use your skin to feel or detect the opponent's strength and intention of movement. This is the best way to get to know your opponent and yourself which may create an opportunity to defeat your opponent. In order to maintain sticking with your opponent it requires you to follow your opponent's movements smoothly without using strong stiff strength against it until you detect a weakness or bad posture. It is at this moment when an attack or defense movement with energy release is going to have maximum impact.

Solid and Empty: This is a perfect sample of using the principle of Yin and Yang. Empty is considered as Yin and Solid is considered as Yang. In the movements when you put your physical weight mostly on one leg or there is real intension of attack it is called Yang. Where there is less weight on one leg or a false intention of attack it is called Yin i.e. Opponent uses right hand and pushes your left shoulder. You decide to use empty Yin to follow the push. You simultaneously rotate your body with the push, combining Yang/Solid on your right shoulder to follow through for attack. Yin/Yang are simultaneously present at all times. During Push Hands you should always be highly alert and use your intelligence to play with your opponents. By constantly changing the Solid and Empty states of the movements it makes it difficult for your opponents to find out where your real intention or weight is and lose track of you. This brings you even more opportunities to win the game during Push Hands.

Skills and Strength: Tai Chi is an intelligent self-defense system and requires more skill than brute physical strength. Tai Chi attempts to use less strength to skillfully overcome strong strength, like a matador skillfully evading a bulls attack. Tai Chi attempts to lead a persons line of strength or attack to a safe empty place (where you will not be hurt!) then use that momentum, along with your energy release to throw or push the opponent even further down that line of attack e.g. somebody wants to shoulder charge a door open. At the last second you open the door. The opponent meets no resistance, whereby you help them fly through the door even more. Having said all that, it is good to have enough strength within yourself to withstand the initial attack, just in case your skill is not sufficient yet or you meet a higher level Tai Chi practitioner. In cases where the skill levels of the practitioners is equal, strength is the deciding factor. Do not ignore strength training during tai chi practise. It takes years to skillfully throw a much stronger bigger opponent around! When your skill reaches a high enough level, it can seem supernatural to the untrained eye.

Q8: *What is your average day of training, teaching and work?*

A: I train whenever I can throughout the day on a flexible basis, having no set time. Sometimes I will go to bed at 2am in the morning and get up seven hours later at 9am. Then in the day I will work on the computer for the Web site, DVDs and Video production, also doing bookwork and administration if there are no day time classes.

Later I will teach my evening classes, which are always run on a regular time schedule. Between teaching each class I always meditate or hold the Taijiquan stance for a while, which makes me feel full of energy.

The training I do usually lasts for around two to three hours at a time. Starting with warm ups, silk reeling and stance practice, then the new frame of 83 form and Cannon Fist. I follow this with the straight sword form which I always practice with or without the sword in my hand, depending on if I have it with me or not.

Finally, Fajing (energy release), stance holding and meditation. After sweating so much I usually have a short rest then go for a shower to help me freshen up, leaving me with a nice feeling all over.

Q9: *Is competition in Push Hands much different to traditional Push Hands? If so, please could you tell us why?*

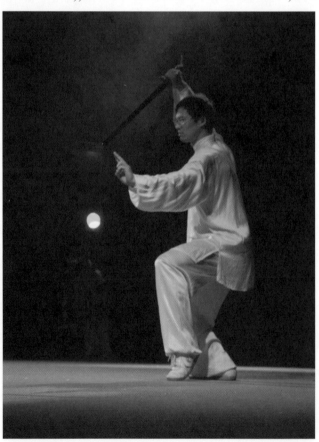

A: Yes, there is a big difference between the two. In competition Push Hands there are many rules for safety reasons, restricting many very effective techniques used in real combat. You have a very limited chance to perform authentic Chen Style Taijiquan Push Hands as it is traditionally supposed to be in the real world. As a result, many powerful Chen Style Taijiquan Push Hands techniques cannot be used as intended.

Push Hands is used as a bridge between form practice and real fighting. Based on sticking skill and body sensitivity. There are many hand, foot and leg movements involved including the eight methods of fighting skill. Which are Ward off, Roll back, Squeeze, Press, Pull, Cross strike, Elbow and Shoulder.

In real traditional Push Hands, energy can be released instantly at any time with any part of your body being able to attack.

Q10: *How do you see Chen Style Tai Chi in the next 30 years?*

A: Thirty years ago Chen Style Tai Chi was only mainly taught in the Chen village and most people did not have the opportunity to train in it. But now they are able to be exposed to the original style of Tai Chi and learn to understand the Yin-Yang balance with soft and hard in unity. The great health benefits are combined with the self-defence skills involved in the form. I think that Chen Style Tai Chi will continue to grow very quickly. Particularly the shorter introductory Tai Chi for Health exercises and 18 Form which help people to learn more easily, which will bring more people in to learn authentic original Taijiquan.

Q11: *What is the difference between Old and New frame?*

A: The original ancient Chen style Tai Chi evolved about 350 years ago and was created by Grandmaster Chen Wangting, of the 9th generation of Chen family.

Old frame (Laojia), originating around 180 years ago, was created by the 14th generation Grandmaster Chen Changxing (Yang Luchan's Master). Old frame (Laojia) is much more simple and more straight forward. There are less twining and circling movements with less martial arts applications shown within the form, such as grasp and arm lock. It is suitable for people who are just starting in Tai Chi and it is much easier to learn.

New frame is an evolving version of the Old frame (Laojia) and is only around 100 years old.

Around 30 years after the Old frame (Laojia) was created, Grandmaster Chen Changxing's son, 15th generation of Chen family, Grandmaster Chen Genyun started to work on his father's Old frame (Laojia) and modified it gradually. Finally he created the new frame with a lot of Silk Reeling Energy twining and twisting movements. Also more applications were added to the form, whereas in the old frame it was hidden and are not so obvious to see. This development process has been carried until the 17th generation, the head and heir, Grandmaster Chen Fake mixed more Qin Na (catching, grasping and arm locks) and modern martial art applications into the new frame, finalizing it. He started to teach it in Beijing and passed on his skill to his students.

The New frame is very comprehensive so it is normally only taught after students have finished the old frame, or to dedicated and hard working students.

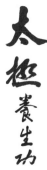

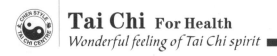

Q12: *You just mentioned ancient Chen Style Taijiquan. What is it?*

A: Ancient Chen Style Taijiquan is based on the ancient Chinese martial arts routines - Chang Quan (Long Fist). The Chang Quan (Long Fist) were created by a very famous martial art Grandmaster, Qi Jiguang, who was a head martial arts general in the Chinese Army. Based on this very powerful and inspired ancient Chang Quan (Long Fist), the founder of Chen Style Tai Chi, Grandmaster Chen Wang Ting, created a series of the Chen Style Tai Chi short sets using an understanding of Yin Yang philosophy mixed with the Taoist breathing techniques.

Each set consists of only a few movements. They are a small combination of techniques practiced with the breathing techniques. Later, all those small sections were linked into the two long series that you see today. The first one is more gentle, soft and smooth. It is considered as the Yin aspect of Tai Chi. The second one is powerful, dynamic, hard and with broken energy releasing movements for martial arts. It is considered as the Yang aspect of Tai Chi and usually has been called Cannon Fist.

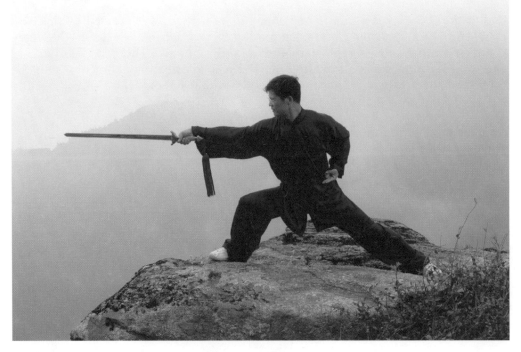

Q13: *Which form do you teach and why?*

A: I teach my senior students the New frame as it is the definitive guide for Chen Style Tai Chi.

I choose the New frame of 83 Form as an overall form to enhance my Tai Chi and Kung Fu skill. For me it shows more real Kung Fu. In the Chen village, Old frame (Laojia) is taught first. Later, only the most dedicated and hard working students will be taught the New frame.

So I choose the New frame, which I feel is the most comprehensive of the Chen Style Tai Chi forms and contains the most exciting and attractive movements to perform and watch. I am happy to say that I have taught over a thousand students the New frame Chen Tai Chi 83 Form. I only teach the Short Form to beginners as it is much easier for people who are just starting Tai Chi exercises.

Q14: *Do you have to wear a Tai Chi suit to train Chen Style Tai Chi?*

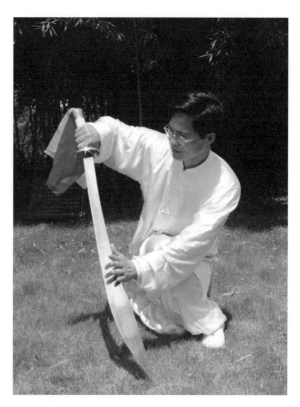

A: The Tai Chi suit is normally very good and usually only worn for demonstration purposes and photographic opportunities.

I have received many phone calls from people asking what they should wear to their Tai Chi classes. I always tell them to wear whatever they feel the most comfortable in provided that it is loose fitting and does not restrict their movements. We have no standard uniform.

To achieve the best benefit from the practice, we recommend that students wear loose comfortable clothes with soft shoes as Tai Chi is a very relaxed, quiet and a soft exercise. A Kung Fu suit is the best clothing to wear for practice and demonstration purposes. However it is only an optional requirement, not always necessary.

Q15: *Does Chen Style Taijiquan work well together when training in any other style of martial arts?*

A: Yes. Chen Style Taijiquan works excellently with any other type of martial arts. I have many students that still do other martial arts styles along side their Tai Chi training. All of them have gained great benefits by adding Tai Chi practice to their existing training. It has helped them a lot and makes them feel more balanced, sensitive and flexible in their movements. In addition, they feel more energetic in their daily life.

Q16: *What is the Foundation Exercise for Chen Style Tai Chi?*

A: The Foundation Exercises for the beginners who have no experience in Tai Chi at all should include:

Warm up exercises - a series of joint relaxing and limb stretching exercises. Qigong & Silk Reeling exercises - Breathing exercises go along with arm spiraling and circling movements.

Tai Chi Stance with breathing exercise - Body standing upright with both arms placed in front of the chest with all body relaxed and using deep breathing technique from your lower abdomen.

Foot Step with Arms co-ordination exercises - Step exercises go with both or single arm exercise in harmony.

Ending with a small set of simple Tai Chi movements which will help you move to a beginner's level.

Q17: *What are the Beginners Exercises for Chen Style Tai Chi?*

A: The beginners exercises are for people who have done some relevant Tai Chi or other martial arts exercises in the past. They should start by learning the 18 Short Form.

The 18 Short Form movements are simple to learn and easy to follow, especially for those people who have done the foundation course or have an appropriate level of martial arts studies experience. It is very easy to learn and to catch up in the classes before you take up the long form studies.

Q18: *Is there any grading system in Tai Chi?*

A: Not traditionally, but there is now a central grading system in China. It is called Duan Wei, in Chinese, and was introduced by the Chinese Wushu (martial arts) Association. In general, this is an optional service provided to Tai Chi practitioners who need it for a particular purpose. The Duan Wei is similar to the Dan system used in the Japanese martial arts system and the highest grade is 9th Duan Wei. 1st to 3rd Duan Wei are lower range grades, normally awarded to dedicated students. 4th to 6th Duan Wei are intermediate grades and normally awarded to the higher skilled martial artists who have been instructors or professionals for years. In particular the 6th Duan Wei holders would have won the national championship in China or equivalent level of skills. 7th to 9th Duan

Wei are the advanced grades and normally awarded to people who are respected experts in the martial arts field with a well known reputation, having contributed to Chinese martial arts development, such as with publications, papers, videos and DVDs. I currently hold a 7th Duan Wei and Grandmaster Chen Zhenglei holds a 8th Duan Wei.

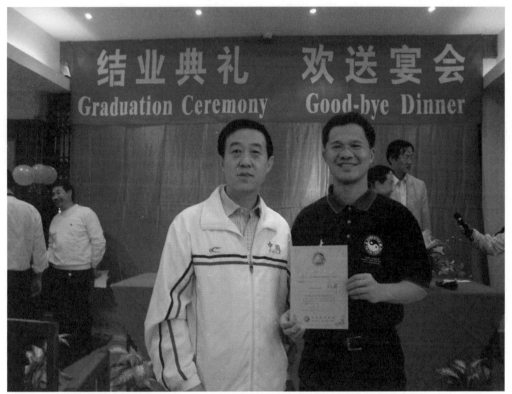

The photography was taken at the ceremony of the first overseas Chinese Duan Wei training and grading course in October 2004 in China.

Q19: *What is Tai Chi?*

A: Tai Chi is a philosophy and is also called Taiji in Chinese mandarin. In theory, it is an ancient Chinese philosophy of Yin and Yang, which comes from the 'Yijing'. Yijing is called 'I Ching' or 'Book of Changes' in the West and has existed over a few thousand years. Basically, Yin and Yang philosophy teaches that everything has an opposite, such as left and right, soft and hard, fast and slow, internal and external, etc...;

The philosophy of Tai Chi was then applied to a series of Chinese Martial Arts movements in the late eighteenth century, which happened to be the Chen family style of fighting in Chenjiagou village, China. The martial movements followed the principles of the 'I Ching'. i.e. the theory of opposing and yet interdependent principles in nature (Yin and Yang).

The full name of what we now see today is Taijiquan i.e. Taji philosophy plus martial arts (and Qigong breathing exercises). Basically somebody had a lot of time on their hands in retirement and a passion for martial arts, producing the wonderful complete martial system that we benefit from today!

Q20: *What is Chen Style Tai Chi?*

A: Modern academics place the origins of Tai Chi in the Chen village in Henan province of mainland China about 350 years ago. Chen Style Tai Chi is practiced both for its health and exercise benefits and as an effective method for self-defense. It can be seen as a series of coordinated movements which flow smoothly and gracefully into each other combined with Qigong breathing techniques and applications. Chen Style Tai Chi is both a complete martial system and a comprehensive form of exercise that promotes fitness, coordination, confidence and relaxation. It is a sequence of dynamic movements that combine soft and hard, with fast and slow actions in a balanced and natural way that adhere to the philosophical Taoist principles of Yin and Yang from the "Yijing" (Book of Changes, Western called I-Ching). Contained within its framework are spiraling, twining, twisting, and unique silk reeling energy movements, jumps, leaps and explosive energy releases. During practice, the body remains relaxed with the practitioner's consciousness, breathing and actions all closely connected. These unique features enhance benefits to health, fitness, and weight-loss and are just a few of the reasons why so many people, regardless of age and level of fitness, regularly practice Chen Style Tai Chi throughout the world today. Chen Style Tai Chi continues to remain true to its original meaning and application since its creation with the current head of the Chen Family, Grandmaster Chen Zhenglei, internationally recognized as one of the highest level masters within the art.

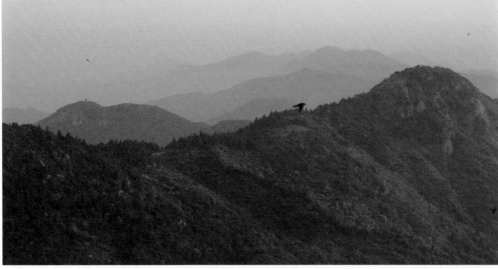

Q21: *What is the relationship between Tai Chi and Health*

A: Tai Chi exercise regulates all systems within the body improving digestion, respiration and also circulation. Since the movements are performed in a relaxed manner, this can also lead to a reduction in stress-related disorders. The low-impact nature of the routines improves the condition of bones, joints and muscles without strain whilst encouraging balance, flexibility and co-ordination to promote health and vitality within the individual.

Tai Chi is recognized by the Chinese Government and many health institutes around the world as the form of exercise that offers one of the greatest all-round health benefits.

Q22: *Who can practice Tai Chi?*

A: Tai Chi is suitable for people of all ages and levels of physical fitness. The movements can be performed slowly and gently in higher postures for health benefits or faster and more powerfully in lower postures for self defense applications and for fitness. The amount of exercise to practice is also totally controlled by the practitioner according to personal fitness levels. No matter how many times you practice a week or how hard you train, as long as you are committed you will gain the great health benefits and enjoyment of Tai Chi.

Q23: *What are the recommended learning procedures for Chen Style Taijiquan?*

A: According to our teaching experiences we would like to suggest the following procedures for beginners to take up in order:

To learn the Hands Forms
Foundation course
11 Short Form
18 Short Form
Old Frame - Laojia

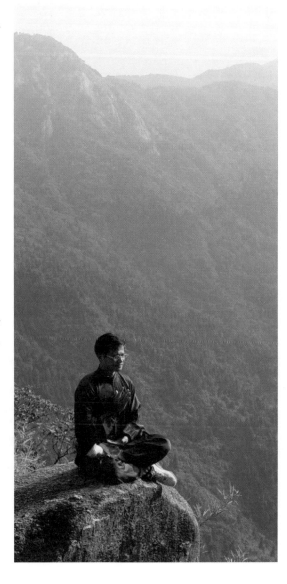

83 Form - New Frame and Laojia Cannon Fist
New Frame Cannon Fist

To learn the Weapons
Sabre
Sword
Long Pole
Halberd
Spear
Double Sabre
Double Sword

To Learn Push Hands and Applications
Single Hand
Double Hands
Moving Steps
Lower Position - Dalu
Free Step
Application - Full contact combat

Q24: *Why does Tai Chi put so much emphasis on relaxation? What is the meaning of proper relaxation? And how can you achieve it when you practice the Tai Chi forms?*

A: Relaxation benefits both health and the ability to perform martial arts. According to ancient traditional Chinese Medicine theory, there are many energy channels running throughout the body. When the channels are free, the energy flows smoothly, the body is in good health and it is hard for sickness or diseases to enter the body. However many people have problems relaxing due to mental stress, poor posture (raised shoulders, over bended knees and tense muscles) and incorrect body movements. If the body is not relaxed, the blockages of the energy channels occur slowing down the energy flow inside the body. This stops the blood circulating freely as well as limiting internal energy.

In order to solve these problems, Chen Style Tai Chi exercises require people to relax their whole body. This can be done by putting every single joint and every part of the body in a specific relaxed position or posture allowing the internal energy to flow freely. The simple example is when you bend your elbows too much the blood circulating through your arm will become weak and less blood will be delivered to the tips of your fingers. Less energy will be flowing through your arm. That is the reason that Tai Ch requires people to bend the arm slightly, only in a rounded circle shape, all the time. The positions and postures in the form were created and tested by the highly skilled Chen family masters in the past based on their own experience from generation to generation. That is why Chen Style Tai Chi puts so much emphasis on relaxation. Particularly, it is important to get the postures and positions altered and fixed with hands-on manipulation by skilled masters in person (in Chinese called Tiao Jia Zhi).

For the Martial Arts, when the body is not relaxed the ability of sensitivity and stamina decrease. A tense body leaves you vulnerable to your opponent's arm lock or releasing energy. If you are tense their Fajing (energy release) can damage you and if you are relaxed you can absorb it more easily. Be relaxed, but not floppy in Tai Chi along with a stress free mental state during application movements. These conditions are necessary to perform high level skills not only in Tai Chi, but any physical sport.

Q25: *Why should you ask for the Tai Chi position or postures to be adjusted with personal manipulation by the masters? Can you learn it from watching a video or reading a book?*

A: The tiny adjustments on your Tai Chi positions or postures by an experienced master make a great difference on the inner effect of your practice. The slightest adjustment can make a huge difference which has to be experienced to be believed. The internal energy increases rapidly followed by a huge amount of heat spreading and flowing all over your body. Your legs will shake and your body will sweat. Those effects are not easy to get from a book or video. You have to attend a class and let the master adjust you in person by hand. These adjustments have to be patiently and consistently repeated until the student can replicate these adjustments for themselves. This takes a lot of time and effort, but will reap great rewards in the long term. It will also unravel the so called mysterious abilities Tai Chi people poses. I will go further to say that this type of training is the key to unlock Chen Style Tai Chi from just being a beautiful form, to being used in real combat. An old Chinese saying goes, "One adjustment by a high level master is worth three years hard training by yourself!" This is why in my class I always encourage students to stay in a fixed position after adjustments to experience it for themselves. Internal Energy and feeling are so difficult to describe and there are many books which attempt to do so. It is much quicker to make the student feel it for themselves, then I do not have to explain it to them. They understand completely by experience, not by reading hundreds of books. I open the door, the student must walk through by themselves.

Q26: *What are the most important issues for people practicing Chen Style Tai Chi?*

A: In general, the following tips are highly recommended to the Tai Chi practitioners:
1). Relaxation
2). Softness balanced with hardness
3). Circling movements
4). Flexibility
5). Quiet and calm
6). Smooth and continuous movements
7). Co-ordination

8). Sensitivity of foot work - "Walk as a cat to catch the mouse".
9). Light body movements
10). Flick movements with elastic and shaking energy release.

Q27: *Does it matter when the arm and shoulder muscles feel sore?*

A: That is fine and is a good sign. It means you have exercised well. You feel pain because the muscles you use in Tai Chi are different from those you use normally. For example, nobody will normally hang their arms in the mid air for as long as you do when practicing Tai Chi exercises. Also nobody will squat down that deep, shifting their weight between two legs. Therefore, different types of muscles are involved during the exercise. It is similar to when you are climbing a mountain and you feel sore muscles afterwards. All I can say is "no pain no gain". As long you can handle the pain, just go for it. The benefits come from hard training and it always comes with a little bit of pain or discomfort (sorry, no short cuts). But the results are great after you keep practicing Chen Style Tai Chi exercises.

Q28: *Is it normal to have both legs shaking and vibrating during the Tai Chi stance when you are only a beginner level?*

A: Yes, it is very normal and an excellent result to come out of your practice. I would like to say congratulations to you, because your internal energy is getting very strong and will start running throughout your body freely. The reason your legs are shaking and vibrating, according to Chinese Medical terms, is similar to acupuncture needle treatment. People who have experienced acupuncture notice similar body reactions caused by the needles. This is the energy running through the channels of a relaxed body during Tai Chi practice. Once the energy flow gets strong enough to run through the acupuncture points and channels within your body, your body shakes less and less. All this with no needles involved, just your body's internal energy.

Q29: *Do you need to practice the energy releasing exercise even if you are just looking for the health benefits of Tai Chi and should you stamp your foot on the floor in the form during the practice?*

A: Yes, it has great benefits for your health. Tai Chi is considered Yin and Yang. The balance and change between the Yin and Yang are the key points of the philosophy of Tai Chi. Any exercises without Yang or missing Yin, are not a complete set of exercises and the benefits will be reduced. The energy releasing movements, in particular, can help your body relax and free all the blockages remaining within your body, as well as making your body more fit. Of course the intensity of the energy releasing will be adjusted according to the individual's level of fitness.

The stamping movements in the form help remove blockages and flushes the Qi energy running over the top of your head, the Baihui point. However, for the beginners and people who have weak knees it is not always suitable at the beginning stages. Gradually build up to stronger energy releases.

Q30: *What are the key requirements for energy releasing?*

A: Energy release is a very important part of the Tai Chi training in Chen Style. It has great benefits for your practice, however there is the potential risk of damaging your body's joints and accidently blocking your internal circulation if you do it incorrectly. So the following are the requirements for practitioners to remember.

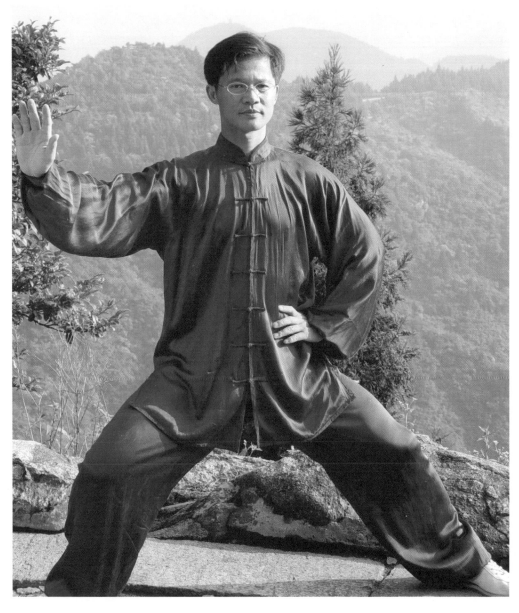

1) Relaxing your body and start with soft and gentle movements.
2) Root yourself on the ground properly.
3) Use your waist as a central axis.
4) Limbs are led by your waist and the strength starts from both feet, passes onto both your legs, then distributes to the shoulder and finally reaches both your fists for the strike through your waist.
5) Free your breath and let it go with your energy releasing at the same time.
6) Do not use stiff strength at all.

Q31: *How long should I stand in the Tai Chi Stance or a fixed position for? Why is there so much pain and discomfort during the practice and how can you get rid of it?*

A: For beginners we recommend that two to five minutes of practice each time should be long enough. Once you get more fit, 15 minutes or half an hour are highly recommended for serious students or Martial Arts purposes. All the Tai Chi Stance or fixed position training always comes with pain and discomfort after you have held the position for a while. Normally you should take it and fight with the pain and discomfort at the beginning stage. Gradually, the pain and soreness will disappear once the level of your fitness and status of your relaxation improves. The more relaxed you are the better your circulation, the more Lactic-acid can be removed away from your pain or sore muscles. Eventually you will feel less pain and be able to stand in low, difficult postures for much longer. There is still pain, but it is bearable, the same as how a long distance runner can keep going much longer than normal people. Again, this takes time and personal effort, like any sport.

Q32: *Do you need to change the speed of the movements when you practice Chen Style Taijiquan?*

A: Yes, it is very necessary to change the speed whilst you practice the Chen Style Taijiquan movements. When the original form was created it was designed under the Yin Yang philosophy, which means everything is based on both the Yin and Yang which changes and complements each other. That is why the Chen Style Tai Chi masters always demonstrate and perform the movements in a speed-change format. The change of the speed varies and purely depends on the person and the circumstances. It is very creative and personal. Another advantage of changing speed is that it makes the practice of Tai Chi exercise more interesting and attractive for demonstration.

Q33: *Is it OK for people with chronic illness, such as arthritic knee and shoulders to practice the Tai Chi exercise and what should they pay attention to?*

A: Yes, it is a good solution to take Tai Chi as a recovery exercise. However, the

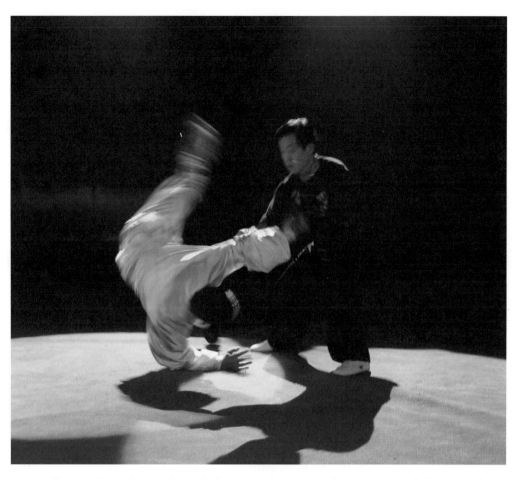

type of exercises, intensity of the exercises and the amount of the practicing time are the main issues to pay attention to. In general, take the soft, slow, light and easy going movements to start with, then gradually practice more and train harder.

Q34: *Where should your eyes look whilst you are practicing Tai Chi exercise?*

A: The eye's movements are very important in Tai Chi practice. The eyes are the window of your mind and it shows your spirit. The following are the key points where your eyes should normally look.
1) Look at the intention, the meaning of the movements.
2) Look sideways using the corner of your eyes with very limited head turning and pay a great attention to the internal feeling inside of your body
3) Look in the direction of the main moving hand.

Q35: *What are the rule and principles of the breathing technique whilst practicing Tai*

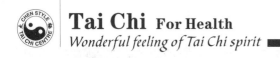

Chi exercise?

A: The breathing technique is one of the main features of Chen Style Tai Chi exercise. Tai Chi uses lower abdomen (Dantian) to breath in and out. Which in turn deepens your breath and enables your internal organs to involve the breathing movements and gain benefits from them.

For beginners just breath in and out naturally, do not strain in any way. Try and use your lower abdomen as this allows for deeper and more efficient breathing, but do not strain . For experienced people the reverse breathing method is recommended, where your lower abdomen goes in and lifts up a bit when you breath in, goes out and sinks down a bit when you breath out.

During the Tai Chi practice, the breaths are always co-operating with the movements simultaneously. It is a very complex training method and it is hard to say exactly where and when you should breath in or out as most of movements in the form can be performed or practiced in various ways or formats depending on the Tai Chi skill of individual and the purpose of using the movements. Therefore, in general, I offer the following tips:

1) Hands rising up, breathing in.
2) Hands sinking down, breathing out.
3) Opening posture, breathing in.
4) Closing posture, breathing out.

Gentle, smooth, deep and long breaths are the main requirements during the Tai Chi exercises. When you practice Tai Chi for health benefits with very soft and gentle exercises you should only use your nose to breathe in and out. When you practice Tai Chi for the purpose of Martial Arts and releasing energy you should use both the nose and mouth at the same time with sound effect.

Q36: *Does Tai Chi have the ability for self-defense apart from the health benefits?*

A: Yes, the original purpose of creating the Tai Chi movements was for self-defense and it has been implemented in wars and self-defense throughout history! The health benefits have just been recognized recently. Many people have recognized the value of the health benefits from all of the Tai Chi practitioners in real life. This is because Tai Chi practitioners are always in very good health and have a long life with a relaxed and happy mind.

Q37: *Why there are so many turning, twining, twisting and spiraling movements remaining in the Chen Style Tai Chi exercise and what are the particular benefits?*
A: 1) Stretching muscles and lengthening tendons creating flexibility in the

joints. It makes your limbs reach further distances and your body become more flexible. The ability of your limbs improves when attacking opponents, and it is also good for defending against arm locks.

2) It twists the muscles and helps with getting rid of fat, and improves the elastic function of your muscles and tendons.

3) All of the turning, twisting and spiraling movements are the foundation to form a spinning motion of defense. It is the perfect reaction against attack from an opponent's powerful strength. Think of Tai Chi as a way of employing an opponent's strength to your advantage, defeating them with little effort. 4) It also helps to remove the blockages in the body.

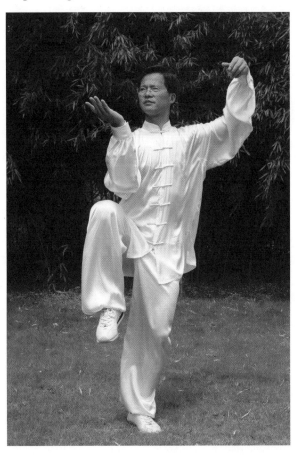

Q38: *Do you need to pay attention to the change of the body's weight and what is the problem if you put the weight or strength equally on both sides of the body?*

A: Yes, it is very necessary to differentiate your weight whilst you are practicing Tai Chi exercise as Tai Chi is the combination of Yin and Yang. The Yin and Yang are always changing and complement each other. More weight or strength is considered as Yang. The opposite, less weight or less strength are considered as Yin. When you shift weight or move strength from one leg to another it can be seen as changing from Yin to Yang or Yang to Yin. If the weight or strength is equal in both legs that shows no Yin and no Yang, it is called Wuji.

Q39: *Does Tai Chi really have functional practical martial art applications? It is so soft and slow...etc. How can you implement the Tai Chi application skill in a real situation? Such as four ounces against one thousand pounds?*

A: I must stress that Tai Chi was invented initially, solely for combat purposes only. In the days before guns, your life and the Chen family's occupation (who were hired for security purposes to protect trade and money transportation across China) depended on your ability to fight. If you had no skill, you could not survive in this dangerous occupation. How could you compete against Shaolin, Wudang, Praying Mantis, Xing Yi, Bagua or all the other martial artists

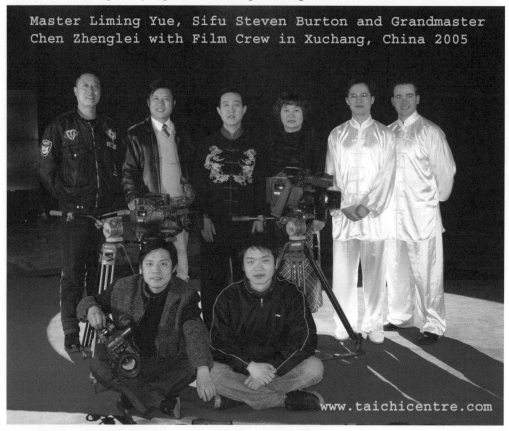

Grandmaster Chen Zhenglei, Master Liming Yue and TV Crew in China during the filming of the instructional DVDs March 2005

with no combat ability? Training for health reasons (other than survival) was not a priority in those days!

Tai Chi movements in general are very slow and soft compared to other types of Martial Arts. It makes many people doubt the ability of Tai Chi to be applied. They think it is so slow, soft, gentle and in a circle, like a dance. How does it work in a fight or competition?

The Chen Style Tai Chi practicing of soft and slow is a unique method of training. It is easy to make your body become completely relaxed, making movements precise and coordinated. Training slowly also allows you to try and combine consciousness with breathing into the movements whilst building up the level of your fitness and sensitivity. Training fast without having trained slow first means you will easily omit all the essential details of the movement. It is just a good step by step training method that ultimately brings efficient and quick results. It is the foundation of high level Tai Chi self defense skill. Without training slowly and soft, you will never be able to produce the fast and powerful energy releases of Tai Chi. This curriculum was realized after much experience in training and teaching by the high level Chen masters. Can you ignore this advice?

In real live combat situations, Tai Chi movements are very fast and powerful. There is nothing slow about it at all. In the Tai Chi fighting song it says, "Your enemy attacks first, but you get him first!" The truth is, speed is essential in combat. I do not know of anybody who can fight slowly.

Q40: *What is the meaning of "bring the opponents in" and then lead them to the "empty place"?*

A: When the opponent attacks you with very strong strength the Tai Chi way to deal with this situation is to never use strength against your opponent to stop his attack. Instead, get in touch with your opponent and use soft contact to stick with your opponent's arm, leg or body first whilst maintaining an effective defense line with minimum strength needed. Once you touch the opponent's attack movements, try to use the sensation of your skin to listen to the route of the opponent's strength and follow its intended direction to bring his movement in and lead to a place where your opponent's attack does not affect your safety at all, as if your opponent's attack goes to an empty target.

This is why Tai Chi always allows the attack to come close to your body but use circling movements with soft touching or sticking skill to redirect the strength of your opponent to a useless position or empty place. Again, this takes time to develop.

Q41: *What is the exact meaning of using any parts of the body to implement the Martial Arts application within the Tai Chi movements and how can you be like that?*

A: Tai Chi training requires all parts of the body to be involved in the movements with relaxed internal energy flowing inside the body. Once the energy is full up and the body is relaxed and sensitive, it will be good against the attack and can release the energy in whatever direction the attack takes place. For the high skilled masters, their bodies have been trained to be like a full ball of energy and it looks like an explosion once the energy is released. Every single point of the body should be able to release the energy. That is why the Tai Chi practitioners pay so much attention to relaxation and making the body work as a whole unit.

Q42: *When is a good age to practice Tai Chi exercises?*

A: You can practice Tai Chi exercises at any age. In general, as long as you can walk freely and manage to move your arm and legs, the safe and gentle Tai Chi exercises for health are OK to practice. The youngest child who demonstrated Chen Style Tai Chi form movements on the stage at the International Tai Chi Festival held in China 1999 was only three-and-a-half years old and one of the oldest students who is still alive and practicing Chen Style Tai Chi in the UK is 108-years old.

Q43: *Do you need to use the punch bag and practice weight lifting as complementary training for Tai Chi exercise?*

A: It is not necessary, but weight training can be a complement . The Tai Chi training system can do it all.

Tai Chi usually touches the opponent first by sticking to the body of the opponent then taking control, before energy release. So, in most of the strikes you are actually already touching the opponent, before releasing energy from a short distance. That type of energy release does not require you to train your knuckles on a hard surface or repeatedly hit your fist or palm on punch bags. Tai Chi energy is always penetrating into the opponent's body and not just superficial damage. The highest level is when the opponent's surface is unblemished, but everything inside the body is damaged. You touch the opponent first then release energy with an one inch punch strike (like Bruce Lee's famous one inch punch). This type of energy release is very powerful but also very protective of your hand, muscle, tendons and bone joints.

Some hard training practitioners may eventually use weight training and the punch bags. It has obvious benefits, but is not necessary in Chen Style Tai Chi. Most high level Tai Chi masters have very soft hands. Tai Chi training ensures that your hands will not suffer from arthritis, stiff fingers and poor finger sensitivity which is very likely through hard conditioning training. So I acknowledge hard training, but do not encourage it. In the past people trained for survival, even if it meant damaging your limbs in the long run! In modern times, this training is rarely necessary.

Q44: *The living room space is limited, how can you practice Tai Chi regularly at home for the convenience?*

A: The amount of space needed for Tai Chi practice is very small. Basically, you need a space where you can walk two steps forward and three steps across. That space should be big enough to practice Tai Chi. The movements in the form can be altered accordingly to the available space you have, particularly for the Eleven Short Form created by myself.

Q45: *Why is there so much emphasis placed on form practices in Taijiquan and why are they so long?*

A: When Taijiquan was created, it was not only just for health but also as a self-defense skill. The form gives you a unique series of individual movements for Martial Arts and self-defense training. All movements in the Form have their own meaning and applications. It is a full collection of useful and practical Martial Arts movements which have been linked smoothly and logically under the principle of Tai Chi philosophy. This offers a daily training programme of comprehensive exercises. It includes stances, hand form, footwork, body exercise and spiritual training. Yin-Yang principles and internal spiraling energy have been used in all of these exercises. People need to practice repeatedly as much as possible to improve their movements and get to know the hidden meaning of the movements. The form is the physical blueprint the masters passed down so the next generation would not lose what was learnt. It is a lifelong journey of practice to enable you to reach the highest levels of Taijiquan.

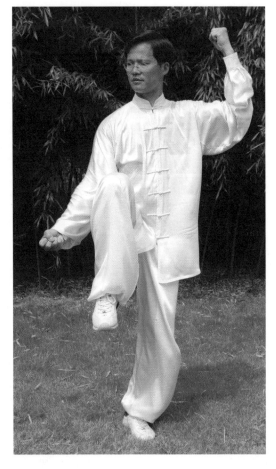

Q46: *When can I graduate in Tai Chi ?*

A: Tai Chi is life long exercise to learn and practice. People work on one layer to another layer and never end the journey of study. So "keep going and never stop" would be the answer to graduating in Tai Chi.

Q47: *Is Tai Chi suitable for kids to take up as a general exercise?*

A: Yes, It is a very good exercises for kids to take up as it helps kids to calm down and be more self-controled. It encourages self-discipline, patience, balance, co-ordination and a high level of fitness. However the type of training methods applied to the kids are slightly different to normal adult classes. We normally start with the hard and fast exercises to keep their interest, while mixing with soft and slow movements in between.

Q48: *What is the Tai Chi Well-being exercises about and how does it work?*

A: The Tai Chi Well-being exercises is specially set out and designed for those companies, colleges and government departments who wish to host an introductory taster session or away day for members of staff to relax and de-stress. It is very easy for people to participate in the exercises and very effective as well. We had very good positive feed back from various organizations in the past. It is a set of Tai Chi Foundation exercises covering Warm Up exercises, Hands with Foot Step exercises, Qigong Breathing exercises, Tai Chi stance and simple form exercises. All exercises together take about 40-50 minutes to finish and it is very easy to follow the instructor during the sessions, with no experience required at all. These are perfect exercises to help people have a break during the middle of a hard working day and recharge the body.

Q49: *Why do the movements seem different when performed by different masters? How does it affect the practice and how should students cope with it?*

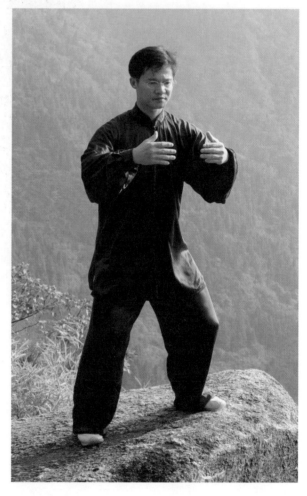

A: Each movement in the form had a lot of application meaning when it was designed initially. By default, when you break the movement down into applications, the ways of practice are obviously different. Also different people have different body shapes and individual preferences, which result in performing the same movement in slightly different ways. This is analogous to one mother having 10 sons and they are all different. So once you put the application meaning and personal preferences together you can imagine how different it could be. However, whatever changes or differences of format of movement there are, the central core principle of the movement always stays the same. Once you understand the multiple applications possible from each movement and figure out your individual preferences, everything will become very clear and simple. Eventually, you can even form your own individual style or way to practice.

As you progress your movements will be performed differently. With experience, the movements naturally become more detailed and your consciousness, breathing and spirit will be built into the form, along with stronger internal energy. Beginners follow the outward frame of the movements in a very big and square way. As you get more experienced you will follow the feeling of the internal energy and practice with more precision. The movements will become smaller and more circular.

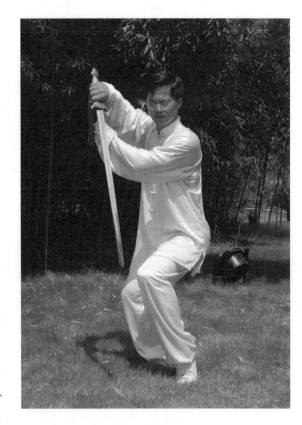

At different stages, even for the same person, the movements will be different. This is the same for all levels and even Grandmasters, everybody has their own personal way of performing Tai Chi, but the principles of the movements always stays the same.

Q50: *What should I do when I practice at home but forget the movements?*

A: The best way to is just try to practice as much as you can remember from the classes and ignore the forgotten bit of the movement. As the teaching session is a coutinuous activity you will have plenty of opportunities to catch up on the details later on. In other words, the benefits of Tai Chi is not from the individual movement but from continuous and dedicated practice. As long as you practice the exercises you will definitely receive great benefits.

Alternatively, the intructional DVDs and Videos that accompany this book would be another solution. They should remind you and refresh your mind enabling you to catch up on the bits you have missed or forgotten.

The end of the dialogues

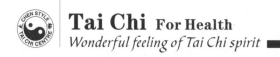
Chapter Eight
Biography of the Authors

Biography of Grandmaster Chen Zhenglei

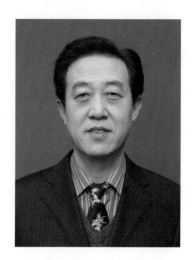

Grandmaster Chen Zhenglei was born in May 1949 at the birth place of Tai Chi - Chenjiagou Village, Wenxian County, Henan Province, China. He is the 19th generation inheritor of the Chen family and 11th generation direct-line successor of Chen Style Taijiquan. He has held the position of Head Instructor and Principal of Chen Village Taijiquan School, Head Instructor of Wen County Taijiquan Promotion and Development Centre and Vice Director of Henan Province Martial Arts Administration.

He has been officially recognized as one of the Top Ten Foremost Martial Artists by the Chinese State Government and has been awarded the honor of National Martial Arts Senior Instructor holding of 8th Duan Wei of Chinese Wushu (Martial Arts) Grading System. He is also a Committee Member of China Physical Culture & Science Institute.

He has recently established the Chen Zhenglei Tai Chi Culture Co. Ltd. in Zhengzhou City, Henan Province, China to promote Chen Style Tai Chi and help the Tai Chi practitioner worldwide to access his unique training skills. Anyone taking part in his training courses will have the opportunity to learn directly from one of the most skillful Tai Chi Grandmasters in the world.

As part of his Tai Chi life Grandmaster Chen Zhenglei has been invited to visit and teach Tai Chi in nearly 30 countries and has published many books and a series of Videos, VCD and DVDs on Tai Chi by the Chinese State Sports and Education Publishing House. It includes Tai Chi Qigong, Silk Reeling Energy, Warm up Exercises, Forms, Weapons, Push Hands and Applications. Many of those publications have also been translated into other languages such as English, French, Japanese, Korean, Spanish.

Grandmaster Chen has been studying Chen Style Tai Chi Old Frame since he was eight years old with his older uncle, Grandmaster Chen Zhaopi, until 1972 when Grandmaster Chen Zhaopi passed away. Grandmaster Chen Zhaopi was a Martial Arts Professor in Nanjing Martial Arts Academy until he retired in 1957.

Grandmaster Chen Zhenglei then has carried on to study Chen Style Tai Chi New Frame with his young uncle, Grandmaster Chen Zhaokui, who was the son of Grandmaster Chen Fake. He was so dedicated to work on the goal of achieving the highest level of Tai Chi that he studied extremely hard and put a lot of effort into his training.

He started to take part in competitions from 1974 and by the end of 1987 he had won over ten gold medals in Henan Province and China National Martial Arts Competitions.

Because of his great success and excellent skill, he has held the position of Senior Instructor at the Henan Provincial Martial Arts Academy since 1983. Under his successful unique training method his students have taken part in the China National Martial Arts Competitions and won 15 gold medals and 12 silver medals over two years in 1988 and 1989, which is a really good outcome. Not only that, he himself has taught thousands of students worldwide to let more and more people enjoy the authentic Chen Style Tai Chi exercises.

Biography of Master Liming Yue

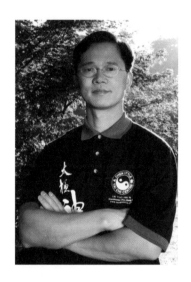

Master Liming Yue originally began the study of Shaolin martial arts as a child in China in 1972. Eleven years later, amazed by the skills of a young student from the famous village of Chenjiagou he began his journey to understand the internal arts by studying orthodox Chen Style Tai Chi under the 11th generation Chen Masters in the village.

Having learnt from the most skillful and experienced Tai Chi masters in China and having extensively studied Internal Qigong with masters from the monastery on Nanyue Mountain, Master Yue moved from mainland China to the United Kingdom and founded the Chen Style Tai Chi Centre in Manchester in 1995.

Since 1982, Master Liming Yue has helped many students to begin a journey of their own and he now spends his time teaching seminars and training instructors throughout Europe, and producing instructional Books, DVDs and Videos. Through his teaching, Master Yue has helped to develop a deeper understanding of the principles and philosophy of Tai Chi that is accessible and valuable to all students and scholars.

In addition to his work for the Centre, Master Liming Yue also teaches Tai Chi skills for Age Concern, the Workers Education Association, and the Manchester City Council Adult Education Service and previously was a part time Tai Chi lecturer for the University of Salford. Master Liming Yue is officially awarded the 7th Duan Wei by Chinese Wushu (Martial Arts) Association China.

Biography of Tim Birch

Tim Birch is an experienced freelance journalist. During the past decade he has been retained by Greater Manchester Newspapers Ltd while also writing for national newspapers and various magazines.

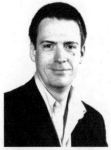

Biography of Danny Chisholm

Principal Instructor: Dan Chisholm
Chen Style Tai Chi Centre - South East Region
Website: www.chentaichi.co.uk ,
E-mail: dan@chentaichi.co.uk

Dan Chisholm is a full-time Tai Chi instructor and Tui Na practitioner based in East Sussex and has studied Chen Style Tai Chi since 1996. Dan is an indoor student of Grandmaster Chen Zhenglei and a senior indoor student of Master Liming Yue.

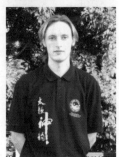

Early in his training Dan spent 3 years living in China developing his understanding of Chinese culture and Tai Chi. During this time he began his training in TCM, studying Tui Na techniques from a group of highly experienced blind practitioners.

Biography of Anthony Rushton

Anthony Rushton has over 21 years of experience in Martial Arts and has been studying Chen Style Tai Chi from Master Liming Yue. The founder of Anthony Rushton Internal Kung Fu Association and he also teaches Tai Chi and Kung Fu in Worcester area in the UK and run seminars in other European countries.

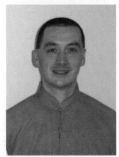

Achieving - Honorary Master of Sha Guozheng Martial Art Academy. Awarded by Headmaster Sha jin jie (son of the late grandmaster Sha Guozheng).

Biography of Nick Taylor

Instructor Nick Taylor - the founder of Devon Tai Chi Centre Having studied under the direct tuition of Master Liming Yue since 1996, Nick is a senior Indoor Student of Master Liming Yue, and has recently been accepted as an Indoor Student of Grandmaster Chen Zhenglei. In 2000 Nick qualified as a Chen

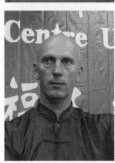

Style Tai Chi Instructor in Chenjiagou, Wen County, Henan Province, China. Nick has also furthered his studies in the U.K., Europe and China with leading Chen Style Tai Chi Masters.

Through 9 years of training Nick has emerged as a talented and dedicated instructor, continuously studying and increasing his knowledge of this ancient art. This understanding of Chinese culture has been complemented with training in Traditional Chinese Medicine (TCM) leading to qualification as a Tui Na Master Practitioner of Chinese Medical Massage, BhTEC ITEC.

Www.devontaichicentre.com; info@devontaichicentre.com

Biography of Bill Wilkinson

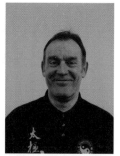

Bill Wilkinson is a senior student of Master Liming Yue and indoor student of Grandmaster Chen Zhenglei, a qualified Chen Style Tai Chi instructor in Blackburn, Lancashire. Bill has been studying Tai Chi with Master Liming Yue for five years and previously with Steve Burton in Accrington. He has complemented his study in the UK with visits to China and seminars in Europe with Grandmaster Chen Zhenglei. Bill is employed as a Senior Manager with Abbey National Bank in the North West England. He is working closely with Master Liming Yue and other senior students to promote the benefits of Tai Chi to Companies and Schools in the UK.

Biography of Shulan Tang

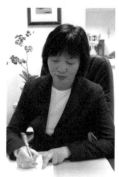

Prof. Shulan Tang, BSc, MSc degrees in Medicine at TCM Universities in China, has held Head practitioner of Shulan Clinics; Managing Director of SHULAN UK LTD; Principle of Shulan College of Chinese Medicine; Lecturer at number of UK Universities with specializing in Gynecology and supervisor at Salford University; Academic Executive of ATCM UK, Fellow member of Register of Chinese Herbal Medicine, UK, Member of the British Acupuncture Council, UK; Prof. Tang has also published 60 articles in a variety of popular and professional journals.

Contact details: www.shulan.uk.com; Tel: +44 (0)161 2279888

Biography of Steven Burton

Steven Burton is an indoor student of Grandmaster Chen Zhenglei and senior indoor student of Master Liming Yue, one of only a few people in the United Kingdom to be certified to teach original Chen Style Tai Chi and certified by Master Jeremy Yau for Lau Gar Kung Fu. He is the founder of Dragon Society School of Chinese Martial Arts.

Gold medallist on Chen Style Tai Chi Form and Silver Medallist on Chen Style Tai Chi Weapons in China August 2004. Five Times British Silver Medallist

Taught and certified in Chen Style Tai Chi by Grandmaster Chen Zhenglei - Henan, China, also Grandmaster Kongjie Gou and Master Liming Yue of the Chen Style Tai Chi Centre UK.

Contact details: http://www.laugar.co.uk

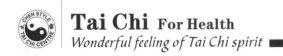
APPENDIX
Catalogue of Chen Style Taijiquan DVDs/Videos/Books/Musics
Online shop: www.shop.taichicentre.com

The Definitive Chen Style Tai Chi DVD & Video by Grandmaster Chen Zhenglei

The Definitive Chen Style Tai Chi Demonstration Video is by Grandmaster Chen Zheng Lei, one of The Top Ten Foremost Martial Artist in China who is considered as one of the best Tai Chi Grandmasters in the world.

The video includes Chen Style Tai Chi Short Form, Long Forms (New Frame, Xinjia and Old Frame, Laojia), Cannon Fist, Sword, Sabre, Double Sabre, Spear, Halberd, Push Hands, Applications and an extract of Tai Chi Festivals. The footage has been filmed over the last five years by the Chen Style Tai Chi Centre UK and all the excellent shows have been collected into this video. It is a really valuable asset for all Tai Chi practitioners regardless of what style.

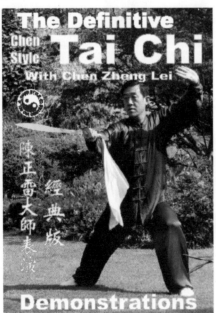

The Tai Chi movements demonstrated by Grandmaster Chen Zhenglei in the video are so graceful, peaceful and powerful whilst the energy releasing is explosive and dynamic.

The movements are clear and precise making this an excellent example of Chen Style Tai Chi demonstrations suitable for both beginners and experienced practitioners. Chen Zhenglei performs the standardized movements as recognized by the State Sports and Education Department of China. This recording makes an excellent reference of Definitive Chen Style Tai Chi.

Tai Chi Silk Reeling Energy DVD

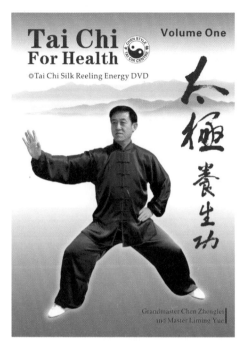

These exercises have been designed for beginners of Chen Style Tai Chi and are a complete health system. It is also part of the book Tai Chi for Health. The video footage was filmed in a professional studio in China with the latest DVD authoring techniques enabling you to navigate and watch the DVD easily and efficiently.

The DVD covers Tai Chi Qigong exercises, Meditation, Silk Reeling exercises and Warm Up exercises. The demonstration of each exercise is repeated from different camera perspectives and at different speeds with detailed commentary to maximize the benefits of practice and implementation.

Tai Chi 18 Short Form DVD

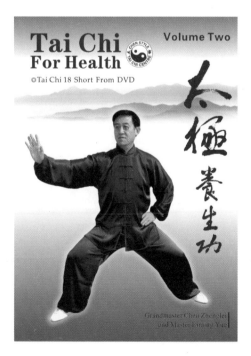

Grandmaster Chen Zhenglei is the foremost authority on Chen Style Tai Chi and the creator of the 18 Short Form. This form has been designed for beginners of Chen Style Tai Chi, and is part of the book Tai Chi for Health. The DVD includes an introduction, followed by a demonstration of the 18 Short Form with step by step instructions for each individual movement as well as explanations and breakdowns repeated from different camera perspectives and at different speeds with detailed commentary to maximize the benefits of practice and implementation. The video footage was filmed in a professional studio in China with the latest DVD authoring techniques enabling you to navigate and watch the DVD easily and efficiently.

Grandmaster Chen Zhenglei Laojia book

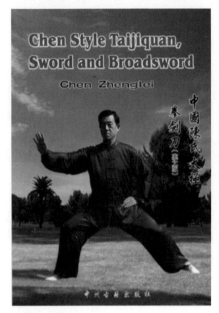

Description:
Written by Grandmaster Chen Zhenglei and translated into English, this new 368 page instructional reference on the Chen Style Old Frame (Laojia), Sword and Broadsword forms is excellent and detailed and offers an insight and depth difficult to find from other sources

Table of Contents
Author's Preface
Chen Wangting and Jiang Fa
The Main Lines of Transmission of Chen Family Taijiquan
The Chen Family code of Ethics
Special Characteristics of Chen Style Taijiquan
Chen Style Requirements
The Method and Progression of Chen Style Taijiquan Training
Hand Forms and Stances of Chen Style Taijiquan
Basic Movements and Chan Si Jin (Silk Reeling Energy) Exercises Standing Meditation Postures
The Fist Routine of Chen Style Laojia Taijiquan
The Name of the 74 Forms (Laojia)
74 Small Forms Divided into 13 Large Forms (after Chen Xin)
The First Routine of Chen Style Laojia Taijiquan
Chen Style Single Sword Routine
Chen Style Taiji Single Broadsword Routine
Afterward
A Brief Biography of Chen Zhenglei
A Brief Introduction to the Translators and Designer
Dedication

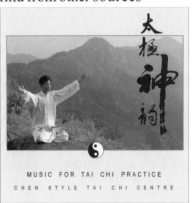

Music CD for Tai Chi Practice

A collection of tradition chinese folk music, recorded in China, that is an excellent accompaniment to practicing Tai Chi. The music contained on this CD is used by our instructors during our classes. We have published the music in response to the many requests from our students. Buy online at www.shop.taichicentre.com

Tai Chi Foundation DVD
by Master Liming Yue

These foundation exercises have been designed for beginners to Chen Style Tai Chi and are a complete health system. It is a follow up (or workout) of simple exercises for people to practice at home or in a gym.

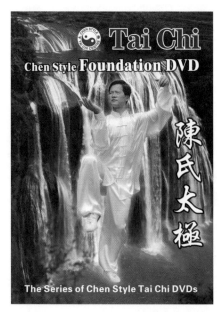

The video footage was filmed in a professional studio in China with the latest DVD authoring techniques enabling you to navigate and watch the DVD easily and efficiently.

The DVD covers introduction, Tai Chi Qigong exercises, Meditation, Silk Reeling exercises, Warm Up exercises and Demonstrations (11 Short Form, Sword, Halberd and 18 Short Form). The demonstration of each foundation exercise is repeated from different camera perspectives and at different speeds with detailed commentary to maximize the benefits of practice and implementation.

Tai Chi 11 Short Form DVD
by Master Liming Yue

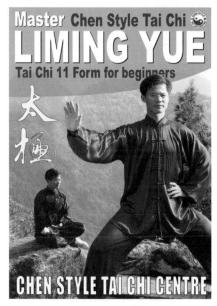

The Tai Chi 11 Short Form was created by Master Liming Yue after many years of study with Grandmaster Chen Zhenglei and Grandmaster Kongjie Gou. The Tai Chi 11 is a simplified form based on the authentic Chen Style Tai Chi Old Frame or Laojia and holds true to all the principles and philosophy of this, the original form of Tai Chi. The Tai Chi 11 is short, easy to follow, and easy to learn, making it excellent for beginners and people who have limited time. Despite its simplicity, the form does not compromise any of the principles that have made the practice of Tai Chi famous throughout the world and can be practiced within a two-by-three steps area comfortably.

It includes an Introduction, Demonstrations (11 Form, Sword, Halberd and 18 Short Form) and Instruction of the 11 Short Form in detailed broken down movements with clear commentary.

Annual China Trip
Sightseeing, Entertainment and Training

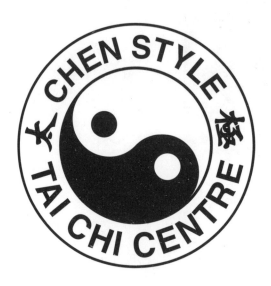

Chen Style Tai Chi Centre

PO Box 137, Manchester, UK, Postcode: M60 1WL

Tel: +44 (0) 161 2737138; Fax: +44 (0) 161 2744967

Web site: www.taichicentre.com

E-mail: info@www.taichicentre.com

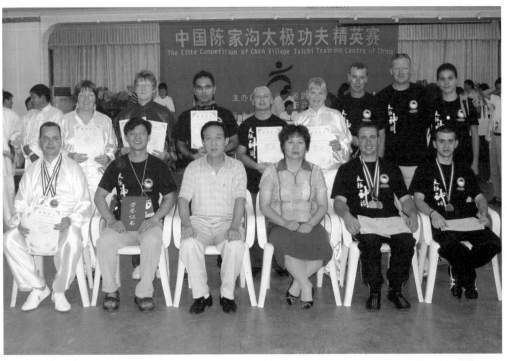

Group picture with Grandmaster Chen Zhenglei at the end of the competition hosted by Chenjiagou Taijiquan Centre in Zhengzhou, China 2004.

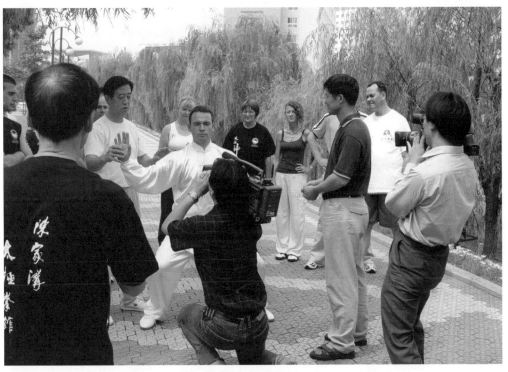

Individual instruction given to the students from Chen Style Tai Chi Centre UK by Grandmaster Chen Zhenglei during the trip in 2004.

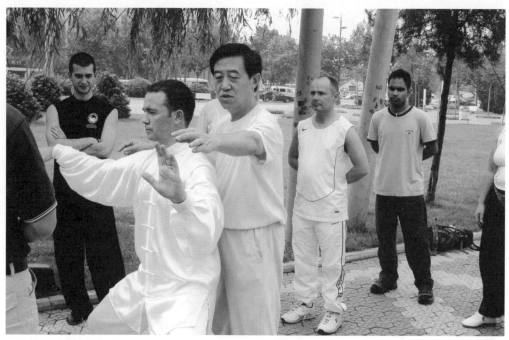

Postural corrections or Tiaojiazhi are the unique training method used in the Tai Chi village.

Introduce to China Trip

The trip is open to all Tai Chi students and friends to develop a greater understanding of this wonderful art with some of the highest level masters in China. As part of the China trip there will be:

A few days in Beijing visiting many of the incredible attractions including; the Great Wall of China, Temple of Heaven, Summer Palace, Tiananmen Square and the amazing Forbidden City. Evening entertainment will include performances of Beijing Opera and Chinese Circus.

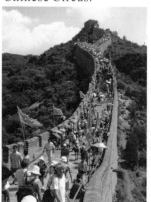

Great wall at Badaling on the outskirts of Beijing

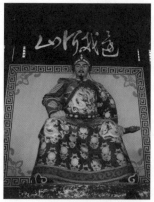

Statue of General Yue Fei – Ancestor of Master Liming Yue

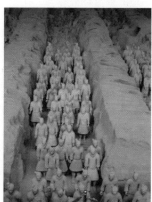

Terracotta Army in Xian

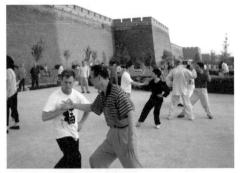

Practice with local Tai Chi people outside the city wall in Xian

A few days International Tai Chi Festival in Jiaozhuo City, Henan Province; this includes entrance to the opening ceremony and access to all competitions. There will be plenty of opportunities during the festival to meet and train with many Chinese Tai Chi and Kung-Fu students bringing with it excellent photo opportunities for all.

A series of training with Master Liming Yue and Masters from the Shaolin Martial Arts School. Students will receive a certificate from Master Liming Yue following completion of the training and will also be eligible for assessment and instructor certification by the Shaolin Martial Arts School and Chenjiagou Tai Chi Centre. (Examination fees are not included in the China Trip price).

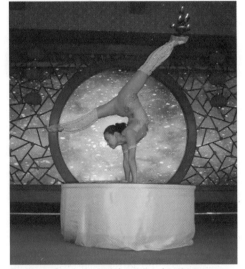

Beijing Opera and Acrobatic show

There will also be an optional training with Grandmaster Chen Zhenglei, head of the Chen family and recognized by the Chinese government as one of the top10 foremost martial artists of present China. A visit to the famous Chenjiagou, Chen Tai Chi village, the birthplace of Tai Chi.

One day training with the monks at the Shaolin Temple including an overnight stay in the temple and morning meditation with the monks.

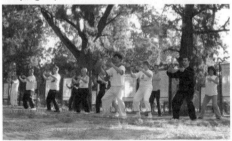

Morning practice in the park

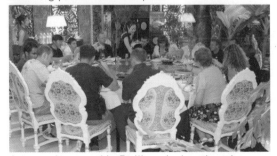

An evening meal in Beijing during the trip.

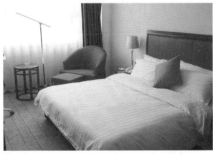

Typical hotel room during the trip.

Details of the China Trip

Date of Trip: 18 days trip over the summer (Departure date to be confirmed). Payment of Trip: Deposit will be required with the application form and the remaining balance of the trip can be paid by installments. The last installment should be paid 60 days prior to the departure date.

Insurance: General insurance for travel and martial arts training will be provided under the cost of the trip (excludes Push Hands competitions). Anybody who is not covered under this general insurance certificate (due to age or medical condition or living outside the UK) will be required to provide their own insurance at their own expense.

Visa Application: Two passport sized photographs will be required for the visa application. These are to be supplied to the Centre with a completed visa form. (Excludes clients living outside the UK)

Departure & Arrival:
Students will be able to fly from their nearest available airport depending on their geographic location. This is likely to be Manchester or London Heathrow. All Flights will be to Beijing International Airport.

Hotel: All hotels during the trip will be of 4-Star standard with typical facilities including: on-suite shower and bath, hair dryer, TV, *internet access, *telephone, *refrigerator with mini bar and *safety deposit box. (*Additional charges may apply).

Rooms are for two people sharing (twin room or double bed). A single supplement is available upon request

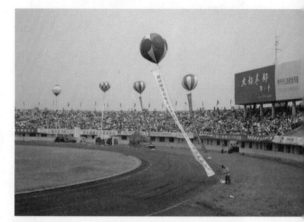

Tai Chi Festival opening ceremony 2000

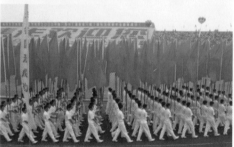

Tai Chi Festival opening ceremony 2000

Top mo

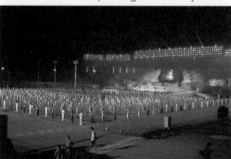

Tai Chi Festival opening ceremony 2002

Pagoda

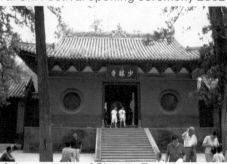

Main entrance of Shaolin Temple

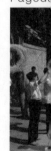

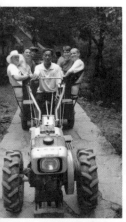
ansportation in China

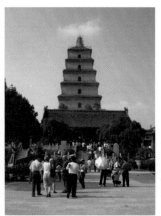
Wild Goose Tower in Xian

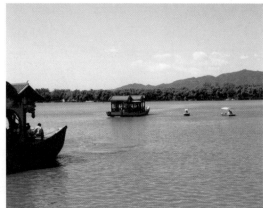
Relaxing on the boat in the lake at Summer Palace, Beijing.

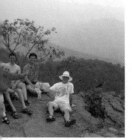
Shaolin Temple

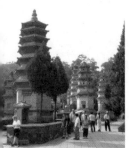
n Temple

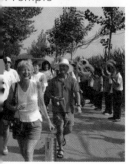

at additional cost.

Transportation: All coaches used during the trip are air-conditioned and of typical western standard. Train journeys are with sleep bed.

Meals: All meals are provided during the trip with plenty of fantastic local Chinese delights including many varieties of meat and vegetable dishes suitable for everyone on the trip. Soft drinks supplied during the meals are included in the price of the trip. Personal requests for specialty dishes and alcohol are excluded in the price of the trip.

Money: Most expenses are covered by the cost of the Trip. However you will need some cash for personal purchases for gifts and entertainment. English currency or travelers cheque should be taken with you to exchange whilst traveling. Credit cards are accepted in some locations (Beijing) but many areas do not have these facilities, so be warned.

Shopping: There will be many opportunities to buy gifts, etc. during the trip as everything is cheap and of good quality - but please be aware of the weight restriction for your return flight. Shipping & Post can be difficult and expensive with many products due to government restrictions. The best advise is take an empty suitcase with limited personal belongings and gradually fill it during the trip.

Training: We will arrange training throughout the trip with much of the intensive training held locally to the Tai Chi Festival.

Competition & performance: Everybody is welcome to take part in the Tai Chi Festival Form competition and performance at an additional cost.

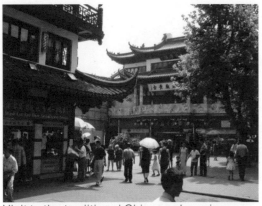

Visit to the traditional Chinese shopping Centre in Shanghai.

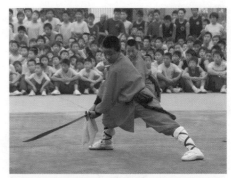

Demonstration by the Monks

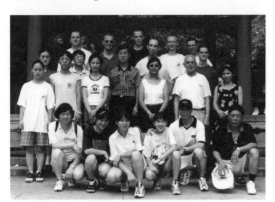

First China Trip in 1997 (below) and second China Trip in 1998 (above).

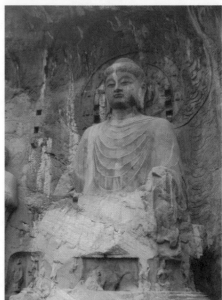

Historic Buddha cave in Luoyang city

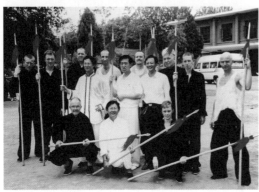

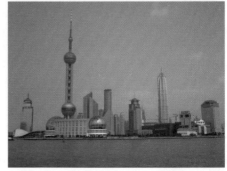

View of modern Shanghai City.

Personal Assistance: Whilst you are on the trip if you need a local interpreter or guidance in making purchases or to participate in personal activities that fall beyond the scope of the trip we can arrange for you at an additional charge.

Certification: There will be many opportunities to receive certification during the trip; competitions, instructor and grading certificates issued by some of the leading Chinese Martial Art organizations plus a China Trip Attendance Certificate issued by the Chen Style Tai Chi Centre U.K.. Please bring plenty of photographs for those certificates.

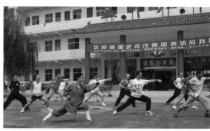
Training with Shaolin Master Geng Jun.

Trip T-shirt: Two T-shirts will be provided by the Chen Style Tai Chi Centre free of charge. The colours available are white, red and black. Please indicate size and colour preference.

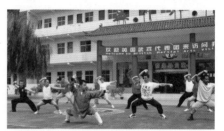
Training with Shaolin Master Geng Jun.

Entertainment: Throughout the trip you will have the opportunity to relax and unwind after a hard days training with Chinese massage (feet or fullbody), Jacuzzi, Sauna and Spa, or even experience an authentic treatment of traditional Chinese medicine including diagnosis and healthcare advice. During the evening you will have the chance to eat in some of the most luxurious restaurants in China, go out partying and perform Karoke. All of the above are optional activities and will be at the individuals expense.

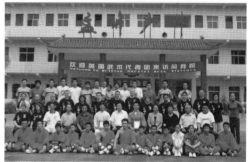
Group photo with the Mengzhou Shaolin Martial Arts school during the China Trip 2004. www.mzshaolin.com

Health Warning: It is recommended that nobody should drink the tap water during the trip. Bottle water is readily available (at low cost) and is highly recommended. Individual activities (such as individual tours or personal appointments etc) are allowed but please report to the trip leader prior to leaving (all such activities are at your own risk). Please take care of your own passport and all personal belongs during the trip. The Centre cannot be held responsible for any losses incurred and special care should be taken to ensure all travel documentation is kept safe place at all times.

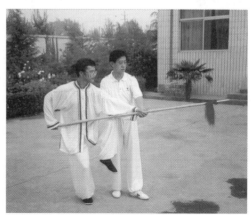
Spear learning with Grandmaster Chen Zhenglei in 1997

Other requirements: Activities such as learning Chinese calligraphy or painting will be a available by request in advance with separate charge applied.

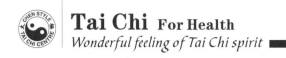

Chen Zhenglei Taijiquan Culture Ltd.

Also trading as Chenjiagou Village Tai Chi Center of China

Authentic Tai Chi Martial Arts
Excellent Teaching facilities and instructors
Deep and vast knowledge of Culture and Art

Chenjiagou Tai Chi Centre (originally Henan Tai Chi Health Training Centre) is a legally registered Centre under the administration of Henan Chen Zhenglei Taijiquan Culture Ltd.

The head of Chenjiagou Tai Chi Centre is Grandmaster Chen Zhenglei, 19th generation of the Chen family in Chenjiagou village, Wenxian County, Henan Province (the birth-place of Taijiquan) and 11th generation successor of Chen Style Tai Chi .

The instructors at the Chenjiagou Tai Chi Centre are outstanding and personally led by Grandmaster Chen Zhenglei, who is one of the "Top Ten Famous Martial Artist" in modern China. The Senior Instructors are Mr. Zhang Dongwu and Mr. Chen Xiaobin, who have won several Tai Chi championships in China.

Chenjiagou Tai Chi Centre was established in 2001. It has been developed rapidly under the great support from Tai Chi practitioners and friends worldwide and over 10,000 students have been trained here since it was established. The Centre is often invited to participate in Martial Arts events and to give Tai Chi performances in China and abroad. It also successfully hosted several international intensive training courses. The students from the Centre have won many championships in China and International Tai Chi competitions. Several instructors and senior students have also been invited many times to teach abroad, with some accepting permanent positions. The Centre is well known and is an influence to Tai Chi around the world.

Chenjiagou Tai Chi Centre has a very nice environment and is well equipped with a very strong cultural Chinese atmosphere. There is a culture gallery and a Tai Chi Art corner where students can express and discuss their feelings, experiences and understanding of the practice. There are also over ten precious pictures of Grandmaster Chen Zhenglei with people from around the world. The 600 square meter training hall is large, wide and very bright with comfortable wooden floors and a mirror wall, which creates a wonderful practice environment.

Chenjiagou Tai Chi Centre is located on the South of Wenhua Road, Zhengzhou City. It is in a very good location with convenient access to public transportation, the ideal place for students and all Tai Chi enthusiasts.

The Centre can arrange accommodation and meals for long distance students and visitors upon request. There are three different ranges of accommodation, high quality (luxury), medium quality (standard) and low cost (economic). The classes in the Centre are set for students of different levels but at the same time are very flexible as well. Students can become members or just pay as you go at a daily rate. Additionally, we hold "the International Chen Style Taijiquan Training Course" in ZhengZhou city (the principle city of Henan province) in August every year.

Tai Chi is a Martial Art that works both internally and externally. In the Centre, students are not only asked to perform all the forms and movements accurately, but they are also required to grasp Tai Chi theory and internal energy in order to applying in daily life.

Tai Chi is an amazing flower in the Chinese Martial Arts garden, that is deeply rooted in the rich soil of Chinese traditional art. Researching, developing and promoting this precious Chinese art is the duty of the Centre and everyone who loves Chinese traditional culture.

Contact details:
Address: 7 floor, Wen Hua Jia Yuan Business Tower, 112 Wenhua Road
            Zhengzhou City, Henan, P.R. China
Tel: +86 (0) 371 63219626; Fax: +86 (0) 371 63219625
Web: www.cstjq.com; E-mail: taiji@cstjq.com

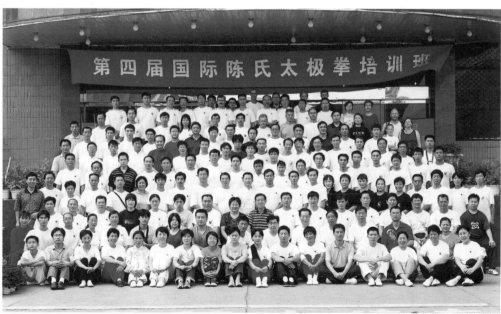
The forth international Chen Style Taijiquan Training course 2002.

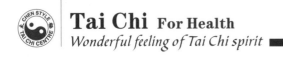

Introduce to Jiaozuo City

Jiaozuo City is located in the northwest region of Henan Province and next to the Taihang Mountains in the north and close to the Yellow River in the south. It includes two cities, four counties and five districts. The total size of the area is 4,071 square kilometers and there is a population of 3.4 million.

Chen Style Taijiquan was created in Chenjiagou village, Wen County, Jiaozuo City nearly 400 years ago. In the past few hundreds years it has been developed and promoted into many other styles by many famous masters. With all the characteristics of Tai Chi such as mixed Yin and Yang, Hard and Soft, Health aspects with Martial Arts application, Chen Style Taijiquan has been spread throughout the world. The Chinese International Tai Chi Exchange Competition in Jiaozuo has created a great opportunity for learning and competing with other Tai Chi practitioners in the world.

Jiaozuo is one of the three highest rice producing areas in China. They also produce four types of worldwide famous medicines, such as Dihuang, Niuqi, Juhua, Shangyue. There is plenty of water and mineral resources. It is a perfect place to develop industrial businesses. The road system is highly developed and is considered some of the best in China. The natural landscape is beautifully preserved and a wonder to see. In Particular the Yuntai Mountains with four sights of interest included in the World Geology Park. It hides ancient architecture built in the Shang Dynasty and is the hometown of many famous historic people such as Shimayi, Hanyu etc. There are six places in total in Jiaozuo city that have been classified as having the highest national level for a preserved cultural asset.

Jiaozuo city was founded in 1956 and it has been developed as an advanced, modern and integrated city. Its beginnings were rooted in coal mining from which it prospered. Now it has evolved to contain power, chemical engineering, mechanics, metallurgy, material sciences, medicines, textiles, food and tourism industries. Jiaozuo is a destination for fun and entertainment too, earning the titles Excellent Tourism City in China, national basketball city and Garden City etc...

The International Taijiquan Exchange competition
Jiaozuo City, China

In order to develop Taijiquan culture, promote the international Taijiquan academic exchanges, make new friends and make progress, the bi-annual International Taijiquan Exchange Competition in Jiaozuo city, China will be held in August in Jiaozuo City, Henan Province, China, the birthplace of Chen Style Taijiquan. The competition is organized by the Chinese Wushu

Association, and undertaken by the Henan Provincial Sports Bureau and the City Council of Jiaozuo. During the competition, there will be various activities, such as the grand opening ceremony, Taijiquan contests, lectures on Taijiquan and assessment of papers, performances of different styles of Taijiquan presented by well known Grandmasters. The people in Jiaozuo city are very friendly and hospitable. We will be honored to have your presence along with your team and friends.

Address: The Contest Department of International Taijiquan Exchange Competition, 401 Jiefangzhong Road, Jiaozuo City, Henan Province, P.R. China Postcode: 454002; Telephone: +86 (0)391-3934492 / 3936439 / 3935343 Fax: +86 (0) 391 - 3933192; Email: fxb520cj@sina.com Contact: Ms. Ji Cuiming Mr. Xu Zhaolun

The above information was officially provided by The City Council of Jiaozuo in June 2005. For English speaking countries please feel free to contact the Chen Style Tai Chi Centre UK if you experience difficulties.

Introduce to Chinese Wushu Duan Wei System

Chinese Wushu Duan Wei System was officially introduced and is implemented by the Chinese Wushu Association in China. It is a complete official system of assessing and grading the Chinese Wushu practitioners worldwide.

In order to develop and promote the Chinese Wushu and the Duan Wei System worldwide the Chinese Wushu Association China will hold regular "Grading and Training Courses for the Chinese Wushu Duan Wei System". The courses and grading are open to overseas Wushu practitioners several times a year in a variety of venues in China and abroad if appropriate.

Requirements for applicants of Duan Wei: Those Overseas Chinese and foreign practitioners who love Chinese Wushu and have practiced Wushu for over two years are qualified to apply for the training course and grading.

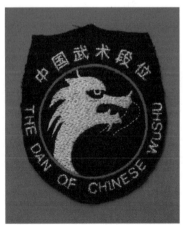

For further details please contact:

Mr. Kang Gewu or Ms Li Xiao Jie
Scientific Research Department
Chinese Wushu Association China
1 Anding Road, Chaoyang District, Beijing City
P.R. China, Postcode: 100101;
Web site: www.wushu.com.cn
Email: wushuxue@sina.com;
Tel: +86 (0)10-64927457
Fax: +86 (0)10-64947202

The logo of Chinese Wushu Duan Wei

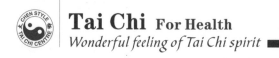

Chen Style Tai Chi Centre UK

Teaching Tai Chi to its full potential

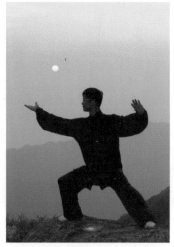

Senior Instructor: Master Liming Yue

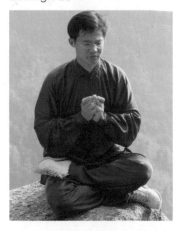

The Chen Style Tai Chi Centre is based in Manchester teaching and promoting the principles and philosophy of authentic Chen Style Tai Chi. The aim of the Centre is to encourage an understanding of all aspects of Tai Chi that is accessible and valuable to all students and scholars throughout the U.K and Europe.

We have three full-time and two part-time instructors, with our senior instructors considered by many as the most highly qualified Tai Chi instructors in the U.K.

The Centre holds regular classes in Manchester and the North West Region teaching the full range of authentic Chen Style Tai Chi routines including; Tai Chi Foundation Exercises, Qigong Breathing Techniques, Silk Reeling Exercises, Hand Forms (11 Short Form, 18 Short Form, 83 Form, Laojia and Cannon Fist), Weapons (Sword, Sabre, Staff, Fan, Halberd, Spear), Push Hands and Applications for students of all levels.

For dedicated students wishing to approach the highest levels, the Centre provides tuition for competition entry and intensive instructor-training programs to become officially certified Chen Style Tai Chi Instructors.

Complimenting the extensive training offered in the U.K. the Centre regularly organizes seminars throughout the world, arranges annual student study trips in Europe and China, and produces a wide range of instructional DVD's, Videos and Books

In addition to the regular adults classes, the Centre also offers a range of classes for children (aged 5+) and can arrange specialised male/female only classes if requested, please contact the Centre for further information.

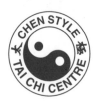

Chen Style Tai Chi Centre
PO Box 137, Manchester, UK, Postcode: M60 1WL
Tel: +44 (0) 161 2737138; Fax: +44 (0) 161 2744967
E-mail: info@www.taichicentre.com;
Web site: www.taichicentre.com